Wellness to

Wellness *to* Wonderful

Praise for *Wellness to Wonderful*

"Drs. Pulde and Lederman have spent years bringing us a scientifically sound and nuanced way of thinking about what we put in our bodies. In this next iteration of their work together, we get critical support for the journey so many of us are on, which extends beyond food and diet: What does it mean to commit fully to a truly healthier and more integrated mind and body? With the gentle and wise expertise we have come to expect from Drs. Pulde and Lederman, this book is the next step to understanding your health and your potential in deeply transformative ways. I can't wait to share this with everyone I know."

—**Mayim Bialik, PhD,** Neuroscientist, Author, Actress, Jeopardy Host

"Matt and Alona have integrated the best of diet and lifestyle to create a whole and complete model of care based on their decades of experience and study. *Wellness to Wonderful* is full of important information if you are committed to improving and sustaining the highest level of health."

—**Dean Ornish, MD,** President and Founder, The Preventive Medicine Research Institute, Clinical Professor of Medicine, UCSF

"Matt and Alona bring to their book an abundance of professional experience and genuine caring for their patients' well-being. Their writing style is relaxed, almost as if we are casually chatting with a friend in our living rooms. Their suggestions of how to navigate the world of wellness, told by professionals, resonate quickly and easily. They make sense, personally and professionally. This book should be in the center of our book collection, at eye level!"

—**T. Colin Campbell, PhD,** Professor Emeritus of Nutritional Biochemistry, Cornell University, Co-Author, *The China Study*, Author, *Whole*, NY Times Best Seller

"No one knows more about the road to total health than Drs. Alona Pulde and Matthew Lederman, and this empowering book brings their knowledge to you. I would encourage you to read it, read it again, put its guidance to work, and share it with those you love."

—**Neal D. Barnard, MD,** FACC, Adjunct Professor of Medicine, George Washington University School of Medicine, President, Physicians Committee Washington, DC

"Simply the best book on Whole Health on the market today. If you have been looking for the pathway to health, vibrancy, joy, and peace, then this book is a must-read. Drs. Matt and Alona weave together a beautiful tapestry of science, psychology, spirituality, and life wisdom that makes every chapter an opportunity to discover the secrets of a wonderful life."

—**Scott Stoll, MD,** Co-founder, Plantrician Project

"I carefully reviewed *Wellness to Wonderful* and found it so helpful that I am going to recommend this as a must-read for all my patients and keep some copies here at my health retreat for my guests to read. It does not merely cover many important issues that are essential to optimal health besides an excellent diet but offers logical and practical solutions to make our lives better—happier and more peaceful and emotionally satisfying. I suggest as you read it, you take notes and write down many action steps on index cards to place around your house to remind you to utilize this wisdom."

—**Joel Fuhrman, MD,** Board Certified Family Physician, President, Nutritional Research Foundation, seven-time NY Times Bestselling Author

"During these challenging times, our nervous systems are bombarded with constant signals of threat. Despite our body's best efforts to achieve balance, dysregulation can lead to extreme stress, overwhelm, lethargy, depression, and more. To thrive in this complex and often confusing and threatening world, it is essential to not only understand this dynamic, but also to learn how to reverse it. *Wellness to Wonderful* provides an impressive, accessible strategy to do just that, optimizing both your health and wellbeing."

—**Stephen W. Porges, PhD,** Author, *The Polyvagal Theory,* Distinguished University Scientist, Founding Director, Traumatic Stress Research Consortium, Kinsey Institute, Indiana University Bloomington, Professor of Psychiatry, University of North Carolina at Chapel Hill

"Alona and Matt understand what it takes to rewire our brains in order to attain our healthiest selves. *Wellness to Wonderful* is truly the ultimate guide to achieving optimal health and wellbeing, written by pioneering doctors who have spent decades in the field of diet and lifestyle medicine. I highly recommend this book, not only to those wanting to reverse chronic pain, but to anyone seeking a wonderful life."

—**Alan Gordon, LCSW**, Executive Director of the Pain Psychology Center, Creator of Pain Reprocessing Therapy, Adjunct Assistant Professor, USC, Co-author, *The Way Out: A Revolutionary, Scientifically Proven Approach to Healing Chronic Pain*

"Alona and Matt are once again pioneering a path to optimal health and wellness. They've taken their years of expertise in the Diet & Lifestyle model and elevated it with a much-needed overhaul. They've masterfully integrated facets of health most of us are not aware vitally need our attention. As the title suggests, their new book challenges readers to not just settle for wellness, but to strive for a life that's truly wonderful."

—**John Mackey**, Co-creator and CEO, Love.Life, Co-founder and former CEO, Whole Foods Market, Bestselling Author

"Having partnered with Matt and Alona as featured physicians in the groundbreaking film *Forks Over Knives*, I can attest to their hunger for and pursuit of uncovering the best and most effective practices for health and wellness. With their new model, WeHeal, and accompanying book *Wellness to Wonderful*, they are once again breaking new ground in health for the rest of us to follow."

—**Brian Wendel**, Founder, Forks Over Knives, Creator and Executive Producer, *Forks Over Knives* documentary

"I began reading *Wellness to Wonderful* as an obligation to old friends. Twenty pages in, I could not believe how incredibly great the book is. I began turning pages as if it were an exciting, well-written spy novel. You will too."

—**Jay Gordon, MD, FAAP**, Author, Member of the AAP Committee on Breastfeeding and Nutrition, Former Senior Fellow of Pediatric Nutrition, Memorial, Sloan-Kettering Medical Center

"What a gift this book is for anyone who wants or needs a shift in the way they feel—both physically and emotionally. WeHeal addresses the myriad needs for our personal health, the health of our community and families, and the health of the planet. The center of this orbit begins with ourselves. Kudos to Matt and Alona for offering new and sustainable ways to optimize wellbeing with a deeper understanding of what it takes to go from *Wellness to Wonderful*."

—**Kathy Freston**, New York Times Bestselling Author, *Quantum Wellness*, *The Lean*, and *Clean Protein*

"In our country's quest to lower medical care costs and increase health and wellness, I can't think of a more prescient book to include in my library than *Wellness to Wonderful*."

—**Dan Buettner**, National Geographic Fellow, #1 New York Times Bestselling Author, *The Blue Zones*

"Alona Pulde and Matthew Lederman have shared a message beyond food. They have created a tapestry of health pillars. These pillars define and enable personal qualities and values which will optimize behavior and relationships, achieving a lifetime of purpose and tranquility."

—**Caldwell B. Esselstyn, Jr., MD**, Author, *Prevent and Reverse Heart Disease*

"Dr. Alona Pulde and Dr. Matt Lederman reveal that although dietary changes can prevent and reverse many chronic illnesses (including diabetes, obesity, and heart disease), there are also cases where diet alone is not the cure. Dr. Pulde and Dr. Lederman show us the bigger picture by addressing emotions, relationships, mindfulness and more to provide a comprehensive approach, so that we will finally have all the tools necessary to achieve the very best in wellness."

—**Chef AJ**, Bestselling Author, Host, *Chef AJ LIVE!*

"Finally! This is the book for which our troubled world has been thirsting for so long—a truly practical and succinct guidebook to wellbeing for the whole being. Whether you are a helping professional or simply aspiring to live your life to the fullest, *Wellness to Wonderful* is a must-have."

—**Paris Williams, PhD**, Director of Centre for Nonviolence and Conscious Living, Author, *Rethinking Madness*

"Good health cannot be fully achieved in isolation. *Wellness to Wonderful* highlights connection and interdependence as integral for thriving. This book is a must-read for anyone desiring not only optimum health but also a wonderful life."

—**Sue Carter, PhD,** Distinguished University Research Scientist, Executive Director, Emerita, The Kinsey Institute

"Alona and Matt expand on their decades of trailblazing in the field of diet and nutrition to provide a comprehensive and practical guide to nourish the whole person: mind, body, and spirit. Seamlessly connecting our relationship to our symptoms, ourselves, and our community, *Wellness to Wonderful* offers a refreshing and compelling look into what makes a life worth living."

—**Christie Uipi, LCSW,** Founder and Executive Director, The Better Mind Center

"The healing journey consists of connecting to every aspect of who you are, gaining confidence by learning skills to process it, and—the most powerful part—moving into your creativity and moving away from your pain. *Wellness to Wonderful* covers these areas well and provides practical information to attain the life you desire. Please don't just read it—use it and thrive."

—**David Hanscom, MD,** Orthopedic Spine Surgeon, Bestselling Author, *Back in Control*

"Matt and Alona have brilliantly woven together a tapestry of factors determining our wellness, happiness, and wonderment. See which pieces of the puzzle you can add to your world and then launch yourself into a more wonderful life!"

—**Rip Esselstyn,** Founder, CEO PlantStrong, Author, *Engine 2 Diet*

"*Wellness to Wonderful* is a bright and comforting message of hope and direction. Alona Pulde and Matthew Lederman chart a course toward your better life by exploring how modern stressors have taken us away from our natural balance. In outlining nine interconnected pillars of life, these noted physicians explain how we must attend to the challenges of balancing work, play, nutrition, sleep, exercise, and authentic social connection if we are to shift our lives in an optimal direction. Written with warmth, empathy, personal anecdotes, and a gentle passion for helping others, *Wellness to Wonderful* is a valuable guide to helping you find the very best of what life may offer."

—**Douglas J. Lisle, PhD,** Co-author, *The Pleasure Trap*

"While there have been many excellent books written on whole food nutrition, *Wellness to Wonderful* is in a league of its own. This book goes beyond the basics of a healthy diet, covering crucial elements of holistic wellness such as physical activity, stress reduction, sleep, play, relationships, and much more. Authors Alona Pulde MD and Matthew Lederman MD have packed this book with practical advice and guidelines, creating a roadmap to transform your health and vitality. They've compiled a comprehensive guide with a focus on achieving sustainable and long-lasting results, and true optimal health. *Wellness to Wonderful* is a must-have for anyone seeking to unlock the full potential of diet and lifestyle to create a happier, more fulfilling life."

—**Jeff Nelson,** Co-founder, VegSource Interactive

"With WeHeal, Alona and Matt have successfully combined supportive healing modalities to make diet and lifestyle changes more attainable for those struggling. I am excited to share *Wellness to Wonderful* with the McDougall community."

—**John McDougall, MD,** Co-founder, The McDougall Program,
    Co-author of thirteen national best-selling books

"If you're a fan of Nonviolent Communication (NVC) or new to this process, this book will support you in integrating the wisdom of NVC in ways that will surprise and delight you. And if you wish to enrich the quality of all areas of your life, this book is for you. It is chock-full of creative and inspirational tools, tips, and strategies which when integrated into your daily practice will surely lead you to what the authors call a state of Life is Wonderful!"

—**Sylvia Haskvitz, MA, RDN,** First Generation CNVC Certified Trainer
    & Assessor, Author, *Eat by Choice, Not by Habit; Practical Skills for
    Creating a Healthy Relationship with Your Body and Food*

"I have known Matt and Alona for eight years. In that time, I have witnessed consistent dedication to living the principles they present in this book in both their personal and professional lives. I trust their deep intention to contribute and the power of connection they transmit in this book. I highly recommend reading this book to anyone who is looking for a holistic and detailed understanding of connection and well-being along with specific and doable strategies for transformation and making life more wonderful!"

—**LaShelle Lowe-Charde,** CNVC Certified Trainer, Founder, Wise Heart

"Drs. Matt Lederman and Alona Pulde are plant-based legends. They understand evidence-based nutrition at the highest level, but now they've elevated their work to include helping people with the true root cause of poor lifestyle habits. This book is a must-read for anyone who wants to truly live their best life in ALL its aspects!"

—**Robby Barbaro, MPH,** New York Times Bestselling Author, *Mastering Diabetes*

"*Wellness to Wonderful* offers a beautifully articulated path for wellness and healing. Taken together, it will change lives."

—**Howard Schubiner, MD,** Clinical Professor, Michigan State University College of Human Medicine, Founder and Director, The Mind-Body Medicine Center at Providence-Providence Park Hospital, Creator, www.UnlearnYourPain.com

"In *Wellness to Wonderful* Drs. Alona Pulde and Matthew Lederman not only share their clinical insights as seasoned medical practitioners and wellness advocates, but also their hard-won wisdom as parents and ecologically-aware, spiritually-awakened human beings. These exemplary physicians offer a practical manual for living a life filled with health, happiness, connection and balance. Follow their advice in this wonderful guide and you can't go wrong."

—**Michael Klaper, MD,** Director, Moving Medicine Forward

"In this genuinely loving book, Drs. Pulde and Lederman elevate the very concept of well-being—and invite you to make that life-altering climb with them, step by step, and hand in hand. By all means, take them up on it!"

—**David L. Katz, MD, MPH,** Past President, American College of Lifestyle Medicine, Founder, CEO, Diet ID, Founder, True Health Initiative, Past President, American College of Lifestyle Medicine, Founding Director (1998-2019), Prevention Research Center, Yale University / Griffin Hospital

Wellness to Wonderful

Alona Pulde, MD
and
Matthew Lederman, MD

WeHeal Publishers
Orlando, FL
support@weheal.health

Cover Design by: Suzanne King
Book and ebook interior design: Booknook.biz

WeHeal Publishers
Orlando, FL
support@weheal.health

ISBN 979-8385773640

Table of Contents

INTRODUCTION

Why Diet Isn't the Whole Picture

"If you want something you've never had, you must be
willing to do something you've never done."
—UNKNOWN

MUCH OF OUR CURRENT audience knows us from our two decades
of work in the nutrition world, starting with a nutrition-centered, concierge medical practice in Los Angeles and branching out
to working on the *Forks Over Knives* documentary, building nutrition- and lifestyle-centered medical and wellness centers and health
plans for Whole Foods Market, and co-authoring five nutrition books,
including a N.Y. Times Best Seller. Over the years, we have made clear
the essential role we believe nutrition plays in preventing and reversing
disease. It is as evident today as it was when we first started practicing
nutrition and lifestyle medicine that a majority of the diseases currently plaguing our society (most notably heart disease, diabetes, high
blood pressure, high cholesterol, and obesity) manifest as a result of the
unhealthy food and lifestyle choices we make.

Addressing the detrimental effects of an unhealthy diet still ranks at
the forefront of our work and our program. But this does not reflect the
entire picture. Although many diseases appear in direct correlation to
our unhealthy food choices, they are also impacted by factors beyond
diet. For example, chronic stress has been shown to increase our risk

1

for heart disease and high blood pressure. Depression and anxiety are associated with diabetes and obesity. Additionally, other concerning conditions such as insomnia, headaches, autoimmune conditions, hormonal imbalances, colitis, gastrointestinal conditions, and mood disorders are equally multifactorial in their origins and exacerbations.

As a result, while nutrition remains fundamental, we have added more to our model. Let's dive a little deeper into why.

Focusing solely on diet, we have helped patients reverse chronic diseases including obesity, diabetes, heart disease, high blood pressure, high cholesterol, autoimmune conditions, colitis, reflux, and other gastrointestinal issues. While healing these chronic diseases was always a huge success, what quickly became apparent was that this was not where the story ended. Instead, some of these patients began manifesting a whole different set of problems that did not seem to respond to dietary changes: insomnia, anxiety, and depression; chronic fatigue; gastrointestinal issues from irritable bowel to reflux to esophageal spasms; chronic pain syndromes including fibromyalgia, sciatica, and back pain; and a variety of random skin disorders.

In addition, we have met many 100% whole food, plant-based people who are physically healthy yet not happy.

In short, unhealthy dietary choices are major contributors to disease, but only part of the problem. For example, according to the Centers for Disease Control (CDC), "more than 50% (of Americans) will be diagnosed with a mental illness or disorder at some point in their lifetime. And one in five children, either currently or at some point during their life, have had a seriously debilitating mental illness."[1]

Suicide is the third leading cause of death for young people. According to the CDC, 14% of all suicides are in people 10-24 years old. Moreover, "in 2019, 9% of high school students reported attempting suicide during the previous year."[2]

In addition, ADHD continues to be a major concern and is on the rise.[3] Children with this diagnosis also frequently struggle with anxiety, depression, and/or mental, emotional, or behavioral disorders.[4]

In short, a health-promoting diet, although essential for achieving optimal health, alone will not cure all ills.

In fact, it turns out that diet is not the only way to impact chronic diseases such as diabetes and high cholesterol. Believe it or not, studies show that patients who had highly empathic doctors had lower LDL (bad cholesterol) and hemoglobin A1c (longer term blood sugars)[5], fewer acute metabolic complications,[6] and lower severity and duration of the common cold.[7] This means that the way a doctor acts with his/her patient affects their biomarkers just as does diet. Even pain was found to be experienced less intensely by patients with empathic doctors. Pain centers in the brain lit up less when a stimulus was given to patients with high-trust relationships with their doctors compared to patients given the *same* stimulus by doctors with low-trust relationships. These are just a few examples of how one person's character can affect the health, including serious physical biomarkers, of another person. We would be remiss to overlook the benefits and additional healing opportunities offered by these discoveries.

One of our biggest challenges as "experts" is to see beyond our own expertise. During our medical training, we learned a common saying: "When you are a hammer, everything looks like a nail." This refers to our comfort with the familiar approach, the one we may know best. The problem is that relying on the same easy solutions often limits our ability to find new ones. We see this over and over again. Meditation experts think the solution to most issues is more meditation and mindfulness. Nutrition experts think the solution to most issues is dietary. Trauma experts think most diseases relate back to trauma. What's more, not only is the etiology of disease siloed by these experts, so is the solution to it. In other words, many trauma experts say that nutrition doesn't matter if you don't deal with the trauma (implying that trauma recovery is what matters most), while nutrition experts say that trauma and meditation don't matter if you don't deal with the food (implying that nutrition is what matters most). Regardless of your expertise, this phenomenon is common and we believe that, rather than merely trying to avoid it, we need to have the humility and self-awareness to acknowledge the existence of this trap of siloed diagnosis and not let it overshadow our ability to see the larger picture. Given the reductionist view of health most practitioners are taught, the only way to see a broader range of issues is to actively look for them.

One of the greatest values we provide at WeHeal, our healing center, is our ability to see the bigger picture and integrate modalities into the most successful healing program. All of the healing modalities we include are powerful in and of themselves, but in concert they have a much greater impact. For example, when your diet is full of processed, disease-promoting foods, then regardless of how much meditation or trauma work you do, you will not achieve optimal health. Similarly, you cannot thrive if you hone your diet but are burning the candle at both ends, not sleeping, not spending time with loved ones, and not making space for self-care.

We believe that one of the greatest impacts we can have on our body is with the food we eat three or more times per day. Equally, we believe one of the greatest impacts we can have on this planet in terms of both protecting the environment and promoting the well-being of animals is through the choices we make with our diet. Our hope with this book is not to dilute the power and effectiveness of a healthy diet, but rather to highlight the additional pillars of optimum health as we define it, getting to a state of Life is Wonderful (explained in Chapter 1).

By assigning diet an important position within (instead of on top of) this paradigm, we don't mean to minimize its importance or dilute the understanding people have regarding the immense impact diet can have on health. Instead, we hope to be able to add to it. It is not "either/ or"; rather, it is "both and." If you don't pay attention to your diet, you will never be able to achieve optimum health, as that is one of the keys to preventing and reversing chronic disease. However, if you focus on diet alone, you also may not achieve optimum health, as there are so many other (non-diet-related) health issues that need to be taken into consideration.

And so, the WeHeal approach continues to highlight the importance of diet, especially when dealing with nutritional diseases such as diabetes, obesity, and ischemic heart disease, but also examines the role of other factors that are essential for healing ailments, pains, and illnesses.

Including connection in our model helps people change how they relate to themselves, to other people in their lives, and to the greater world around them.

The importance of this will be emphasized throughout the book, but the immediate impact and benefit can be seen in a greater tenderness and compassion that all of us can feel toward ourselves. This alone motivates and supports our effort to change. Rather than coming from a place of shame, anger, frustration, and blame, we learn to come from a space of acceptance, patience, and curiosity. In this state of mind, we are more open to learning from our mistakes, rather than repeating them over and over. Additionally, connection helps us heal broken relationships, willingly enhance our contribution to society, and focus on the things we want rather than the things we don't want. The latter is especially important in inspiring us to take better care of ourselves, including eating more healthfully.

One of the greatest contributions we can make as healers is to help clients figure out what is preventing them from making the changes they desire. This book is for all of you who struggle to make long-term and successful dietary and other health-promoting changes. This book is for those of you who can't quite get to a state of Life is Wonderful but want to. This book is for people who have diseases, disorders, or discomforts that remain despite an optimized diet. Maybe you are not as happy as you would like, maybe your connection to your family and friends is lacking, maybe you wake up feeling tired in the morning, maybe you don't have the meaning and purpose in your life that you long for, maybe you forgot how to play or have fun, or maybe you need help learning how to eat better and move more. Regardless of why you are reading this book, we are happy to have your attention. After all, we know that life can truly be wonderful, so please keep reading, as we are confident that we can help you.

CHAPTER 1

Is Your Life Wonderful?

"Your present circumstances don't determine where
you can go. They merely determine where you start."
—NIDO QUBEIN

IS YOUR LIFE WONDERFUL?
You may be asking "when" or "what does that even mean?" Or
maybe you are scoffing at it as a fool's dream—unattainable in real life.

With so many of us living in survival mode, life becomes less of
an experience and more of a job; we are occupied with what we need
to get done, and how we can be more productive and efficient. We are
so busy "doing" that we cannot spend time "being" or feeling. Balance,
happiness, and joy take a back seat to keeping our jobs, paying the rent,
and having enough food.

This makes sense evolutionarily: to evolve we needed to stay alive.
It is therefore no wonder that we focused on the activities that kept us
going, such as eating, drinking, avoiding danger, and procreating. For
further motivation, our brains also released chemicals that made us
feel pleasure whenever we performed these activities. What took priority
was self-preservation and protection, not joy.

We are still programmed to survive, first and foremost. As such, we
continue to scan for danger rather than seek pleasure. It was imperative
that our ancestors saw a saber-toothed tiger in time to successfully run
away from it. For us today, that saber-toothed tiger is largely fear—fear
that we will fail, fear that we will not have enough. How am I going to

pay my mortgage to keep a roof over my head? How am I going to be able to afford to send my kids to college? How am I going to pay all of my bills and put food on the table? How am I going to keep my family safe from all harm? How am I going to get my weight and/or health under control? How am I going to fix my relationships with my kids, my family, or my friends?

When we are consumed by fear, life situations seem fixed. We believe that this is just the way it is and the way it will always be. But the reality is that nothing is permanent. Life is dynamic with ups and downs. A circumstance or situation is just that—one event in time. If we can see it as such, we become players *in* what happens next versus victims *of* what happens next.

Remaining in the fear-based mentality drives the thinking that we need to accumulate more to be secure. More becomes better—we become addicted to more resources, more stuff, more wealth. The more wealth we have, the more worth and status we believe we will have. Erroneously, we think this will bring us the love and safety we seek.

As medical professionals, we have been in the nutrition business for a long time and our best example of this desire for "more" is fear around getting enough protein. Most people don't know how much protein they are getting. Most people don't know how much protein they need. But despite that, they are convinced they are not getting enough and need more.

The cost of this scarcity and fear-based mentality is huge. We define success by having more; we don't know how much more but we know we don't have enough and will be happier if we could just get more. Yet seeking more is a never-ending chore. So we end up in an ongoing chase for happiness with no finish line. Is it any wonder, then, that we are working harder, spending less time on pleasurable activities, neglecting family and friends, yet still miserable in our quest for more?

By mistaking motion for progress, we remain in the daily grind. In essence, we are so distracted with preventing all that we fear from happening in the future that we sacrifice feeling alive in the present.

Consider this example:

Bob was an immigrant to the United States. Wanting to provide a better life for his family, he made himself available whenever work was offered. This resulted in many hours spent at work or thinking about work, including nights and weekends. Bob's perseverance did pay off for his family, affording them many opportunities he never had. His children traveled around the U.S. and got to visit other countries. They played sports and musical instruments, experienced culture and entertainment in a variety of forms, had cars, and were funded through their university years. Bob was busy building a dream life for his family to enjoy. For himself, he vowed that when he retired, he would enjoy the perks of his labor. Tragically, he never made it to retirement, suffering a fatal heart attack at 55.

So many of us live our lives like Bob—we are working for our families, our children, our savings, our retirement. Our hope lies in tomorrow being better than today. When we have enough status and wealth, when our house is big enough, when we have the new car we want, when we finally get enough... then we will be happy. Yet the key to Life Is Wonderful is understanding that it is not about being happy all the time. It's embracing life in its totality, with all of its ups and downs, that can make it wonderful. It's about finding joy even when you are uncertain, uncomfortable, sad, angry, scared, or grieving. The idea is to be intentional about where we place our energy and what we give attention to. Our circumstances may not change but our perception of them can, and in that way, we can make different choices that may impact outcomes. In the words of Dr. Wayne Dyer, "When we change the way we look at things, the things we look at change."[1]

What if our ultimate currency was joy, resulting from a wonderful life, rather than all the stuff and money we accumulate? How could we experience more joy in our lives? And how can we do that in the present, not waiting for it to happen sometime in the future?

We can start by getting out of our heads and into our hearts. Our heads think, analyze, access, interpret, and integrate information; they look to see how to fit all of the pieces into place to keep us surviving. As a result, we scan for danger, we scan for safety, we recall the past to prevent repeating mistakes, and we try to predict the future and guide our behavior accordingly. Our world becomes contracted, smaller, and focused on the strategies that will resist and prevent pain and danger while securing our survival. We lose creativity, openness, trust, and a greater vision of what is possible.

Our hearts, on the other hand, know that when we find joy within, everything else falls into place. The trust here is not in some ethereal magic but rather in the understanding that, when we are happy, we naturally lift ourselves out of a scarcity mentality and become more expansive. This doesn't mean that our troubles go away, or that our struggles disappear. On the contrary, by embracing the unpleasantness of our struggles, we allow them to flow and pass and, over time, we fear and resist them less. In this expansive and accepting space, we are more open to seeing and exploring the many opportunities and choices available to us. And believe it or not, there is an abundance of these opportunities if we only open our eyes to see them.

We may recall a personal story of someone finding happiness and joy after starting anew. Or we may be more familiar with the tale often found in books or movies where the hero becomes disillusioned with their current life and tired of the hamster wheel. At their wit's end, they leave their current life behind to start a new adventure. Along the way, they discover riches far beyond any the material world previously offered them. Among these are new places, friendships, and even love. But above all else is a newfound awakening and self-discovery and, as a consequence, the ultimate currency—a joyous and wonderful life.

So, in a world of endless possibilities, why can't ours be a positive, joyful path? Is there a way to provide for ourselves and our families while also experiencing joy? Can we simultaneously survive AND thrive? Can life truly be wonderful?

At WeHeal, we have redefined optimal health. The measurement has come down to asking yourself, "Is my life wonderful?" If, when you are asked by others, "How are you doing?", you are likely to respond, in effect, "I may have my ups and downs, but overall my life is wonderful!"—then, great, keep doing what you are doing. If you are not likely to respond that way at all, continue reading.

As Nelson Mandela said, "It always seems impossible until it's done."

And it can be done. This is our wish for you and our aim throughout this book… so let's begin making your life wonderful!

CHAPTER 2

Getting Out of Survival Mode

"The trouble with life in the fast lane is that
you get to the end in an awful hurry."
—UNKNOWN

ONE OF THE BIGGEST hurdles to making life wonderful is living in survival mode, lowering our heads and soldiering on day after day, dealing with whatever comes our way as it comes. We know what survival mode looks like at a meta-level. And we know how bad it feels day-in and day-out: the exhaustion, the fear, the dissatisfaction, the desire for something different and more fulfilling.

In survival mode, we develop a scarcity mentality: there is never enough. To increase our chance of survival and to meet our needs for safety, we accumulate resources, we chase after more and better—more money, better jobs, bigger houses, and so forth. "More" seems to wrap us in a false sense of security and protection. It shields us from scarcity and thereby protects us from danger. The problem is that seeking "more" is a race with no end; there can always be more, at least in our minds. So, with all that we may have, we are still left feeling dissatisfied and scared.

Part of our drive for "more" and "better" is our discomfort with discomfort. We have lost resilience, the ability to trust that we will be okay despite adversity. Instead, we try to prevent unpleasant circumstances by trying to control the present and predict the future. Our life becomes something we *manage* while failing to actually *experience*—again leaving us feeling dissatisfied and scared.

What if instead of running away from discomfort, we leaned into it? What could that acceptance look like? Why are people so afraid of discomfort, and especially afraid of experiencing unpleasant emotions?

Many of us have been taught to suppress negative emotions since childhood. We have heard "Turn that frown upside down," or "You don't know how good you have it," or "Don't be such a downer," and the many variations in between. And as a result, we have learned to keep our "negativity" to ourselves. Acceptance is a tender need for many, and a survival need for children. If their parents don't accept them, younger children may literally not survive. So, it is no wonder that we have become so proficient in keeping our negative emotions (the emotions our caregivers or superiors don't condone) locked deep inside. Unfortunately, suppressing these emotions comes at a cost to our overall well-being, including fewer close relationships, lower satisfaction with life, elevated blood pressure, and poor memory.[1]

We need to overcome this default reaction by creating new neural pathways that allow us to not only feel these negative emotions but trust that we will be safe in doing so. Unlike children, most adults are no longer solely dependent on others for their survival. As a result, they have more agency and choice in how they address discomfort. Instead of seeking to avoid the judgment of others by suppressing negative emotions, we as adults can meet our need for acceptance and safety with many other strategies.

Let's start with acceptance. We have found that one of the most effective strategies is a shift from seeking external acceptance to finding internal acceptance. The more we can align with our own values, the more we become empowered and enrich our sense of self-worth. This is hard to do if your entire paradigm was built on seeking external approval from parents, teachers, bosses, and other authority figures. The challenge for most people is to escape the influence of external factors that sway their thinking and behavior. Similar to changing your currency from money to joy (Chapter 1), you can change how you meet your need for acceptance, self-worth, and value by seeking internal over external validation. For example, rather than focusing on whether other people approve of you, you can check in with yourself. Are you showing up as you desire? Are you living in harmony with your values? And if you are, then practice approving of yourself, and letting that be enough.

Once you are comfortable with internal validation, you can move on to safety. Why in this order? It is important for you to believe in yourself and to look to yourself for messages of safety. The world around us is unpredictable and the only thing we truly have control over is ourselves. In practicing self-acceptance, you empower yourself with agency and can use that strength and competence to help yourself feel safe.

Stress is a mental state in which messages of danger overwhelm messages of safety. Living in survival mode, we are constantly scanning for danger, which results in experiencing stress. With repeated occurrences and extended duration, this accumulation of stress becomes chronic. We are not designed to live in chronic survival mode. In fact, our ancestors experienced danger and threat in short bursts. They would see a threat, they would escape from the danger, and then they would rest and recover.

Unfortunately, today the threats we perceive are pervasive and often constant, primarily because they come from our thoughts, not actual physical danger. We are not just running from the tiger, we are raging on the road, worrying about our finances, struggling to balance work and home life, concerned about our children, anxious about the relationships we have or the ones we want and don't yet have, and so on. This threat exists in a mind that, in survival mode, doesn't shut off danger signals. In fact, your body is designed to raise the ante, or in other words, to "see your threat and raise you another threat" that you haven't considered yet, all in an effort to protect you from anything and everything possible while increasing your chances of survival. As a result, we never get to rest or recover and thus our bodies remain in a perpetual state of threat or high alert.

Therefore, a strategy that was once beneficial to our survival has transformed into one that has become detrimental to it. Chronic stress is linked to all sorts of proinflammatory states and conditions, challenges with fertility, and increased risk of asthma, heart disease, obesity, pain (headaches, back and neck pain), gastrointestinal issues (reflux, heartburn, colitis), depression, insomnia, and immune suppression, among other health issues.

Unfortunately, the ups and downs of daily living make it impossible to rid ourselves of stress. Instead, to reach the state of Life Is Wonderful, we need to learn to manage our daily challenges differently. We can do this by giving our bodies messages of safety instead of messages of danger. Here are a few exercises you can try to signal safety and reduce stress.

- Use facial expressions to dampen the threat response and increase your sense of safety. Try singing or humming your favorite tune. Share a smile with someone, even if it is just yourself in the mirror. Studies show that smiling, regardless of whether you are happy or not, can help lower your heart rate and more quickly recover from a stress response.[2]
- Take some deep slow breaths, breathing in for a count of three and out for a count of seven. Slow breathing techniques increase relaxation, alertness, and comfort while decreasing anxiety, depression, confusion, and anger.[3]
- Use your five senses to bring your attention to the present moment, most likely a time when you are indeed safe. This grounding technique helps reduce stress and anxiety by shifting our perception away from danger and towards safety. You can engage with the five senses in several ways. 1) Step outside with a cup of tea (taste), smell a flower (smell), listen to birds chirping (hear), look at the trees around you (see), and feel the weather on your skin (feel). 2) Another variation is the 5-4-3-2-1 technique. Find and name five things you can see (sky, clouds, flowers, butterflies, trees), four things you can feel (wind, warmth, hair on neck, ground), three things you can hear (traffic, talking, birds), two things you can smell (grass, flowers), and one thing you can taste (tea).
- See Appendix A for additional ideas.

CHAPTER 3

The Disconnection Epidemic

"Our survival as a species depends on our ability
to recognize that our well-being and the well-being
of others are in fact one and the same."
—MARSHALL ROSENBERG

IN ADDITION TO LIVING in survival mode and chronic stress, we are experiencing a loneliness epidemic despite being more "connected" than ever through technology. Surprisingly, those who report feeling most alone are people under thirty-five who avidly use social networking and are frequent flyers on their devices. How could it be that with so many "friends" and access to so many people and so much information, we can feel lonelier than we ever have? And is it surprising that in this loneliness we can't experience Life Is Wonderful?

Many of us, young and old, have become addicted to our devices. Even those of us who are not necessarily addicted to them still fall into misusing, overusing, or abusing them. The instant gratification provided by our devices is fuel to the fire and supports our desire to remain plugged in. We have become a people afraid of missing out. And in our efforts to stay in the know, we are losing true connection.

Our currency is once again off the mark as we create social media facades meant to represent our lives. We share (real or imagined) images meant to convey how great our lives are—images of the vacations we go on, the cars we buy, the houses we live in, and so forth. And we look and see how that compares to the lives of our online "friends."

Unfortunately, these are not the experiences or conversations that truly connect. Vulnerability and authenticity have been replaced with false pretenses and fabrications. We invent the life we think we want. The challenges here are numerous and costly. First and foremost, we generate the need to maintain this make-believe image we have created. Keeping up with the Joneses is no longer limited to your neighborhood. Instead, we are now trying to measure up to celebrities. The standard for success and a happy life becomes having what they have, going where they go, and doing what they do. Anything short of that feels like a failure—we are missing out or don't have enough.

Is it any wonder with the bar being set so high that so many of us walk around depressed, anxious, and stressed? And is it at all surprising, when worldwide we are spending an average of seven hours a day online, that we prioritize our connections in that space over meeting in-person?[1]

The reality, however, is that it is the in-person contact that matters the most. According to an online survey of over 10,000 adults, the more in-person connections you have, the lower your loneliness score.[2]

It is our vulnerability, derived from both what is working in our lives and what is not, that provides us with connection to our equally vulnerable friends and family. In these mutually authentic relationships, we discover the people who truly know us, and in that familiarity we find our true sense of safety. We find as well the comfort of knowing that we have someone we can call in an emergency—a person with whom we can let it all hang out: the good, the bad, and the ugly. And relief that there is a place where we can be accepted for being ourselves.

Does this mean that all social media should go out the window? No. However, with the scale being so heavily tipped toward social media engagement, it does require more mindfulness to get back to balance. Remember from Chapter 2 that the stress response is an imbalance between messages of danger and messages of safety. When we immerse ourselves in a world of facades where we can never truly measure up, where we see something we think we need but can't attain, then we are sending ourselves regular signals of danger—not getting something you need feels dangerous. Getting back to balance is therefore key for decreasing the stress response and increasing our sense of security.

As in the story of Goldilocks, the goal becomes about what is just right—not too much and not too little. This extends to sleep, exercise, eating, work-life balance, the use of devices, and all the daily uses of our time. Our opportunity resides in identifying our intention and connecting to our needs with each of these activities. For example, the intention with sleep is to meet needs for rest and regeneration. Two hours is not enough and ten may be too much but seven to eight provides the rest we need and allows us to feel refreshed and ready for the day. Similarly, attaining clarity on intentions and needs allows us to navigate our device rather than succumb to it. Designating a time to check emails sets the intention to meet needs for connection, communication, and information. In this manner, a device is used as a tool for a specific purpose with a set time. This is very different from surfing the internet with no specific intention or need and getting mindlessly lost in the device. The cost here is loss of presence and connection, whether with ourselves or others. When we feel alone and not seen by others, that feels dangerous.

Beyond loneliness, there are additional consequences to disconnection. There is significant evidence correlating a lack of social connections with early death.[3] Disconnection and loneliness have also been shown to increase the risk of heart disease, stroke, dementia, depression, anxiety, and obesity.[4] Our inability to experience and cope with chronic pain is linked to disconnection. In fact, social exclusion and the resulting isolation results in increased sensitivity to pain.[5] It turns out that our rejection (by self or others) physically hurts![6]

We have good news to share. There is a way out of this darkness. There is a path to Life Is Wonderful. The first step is disengaging from our devices. This is not an all-or-nothing proposition and does not mean that your choice is either to be addicted to your device or to throw it away. Instead, we need to find our personal balance and, where we can, tip it toward in-person connections. Start slowly if you need to. Consider a digital hiatus between 8:00 pm – 6:00 am. Use this time to check-in rather than check-out by making this device-free time about connecting with others or enjoying some long-forgotten hobbies. If you are inspired, you can begin or enrich a meditation practice. The opportunities are plentiful, and the only rule is to leave the devices behind.

Devices, however, are not the sole cause of loneliness. We are also hampered by living in a world of facades and by lacking a place where we can be our authentic selves. As a result, the path out of loneliness is through relationships that are authentic and vulnerable, not superficial or phony. We should value quality over quantity—a very different frame of reference from social media where the goal is to amass as many "friends" as possible. One friend with whom you can be your true self may prove their weight in gold as far as contributing to your well-being, decreasing your loneliness, and enhancing the joy you derive from life.

We have found that many experts discuss needing to be authentic or to find your authenticity but then leave you on your own to figure out how to do that. We hope to differentiate ourselves by not only encouraging you to find your authenticity but showing you how to make that shift, even when your body is fighting against it. After all, if your belief is that showing up authentically is dangerous, especially in the face of potential conflict, then why would you risk doing so, regardless of what the experts may say? Nonviolent Communication (NVC), a concept we delve into later in the book, is key to providing a safe space for authentic communication and connection. The NVC skills we will teach you will help you develop agency, confidence, and clear strategies for navigating vulnerability, authenticity, and honesty in relationships.

Initially, these changes may feel uncomfortable. You may experience a strong pull back to the world of devices or solitude. It might feel scary to connect vulnerably and authentically with others. We mentioned above the opportunity to "check-in" despite wanting to "check-out." The idea here is to be mindful of when you desire to "numb-out," and instead of doing so, begin to implement new behaviors that introduce healthy comfort habits over harmful ones that support avoidance and disconnection.

It is ironic that the one thing that trumps our desire to seek pleasure is our drive to avoid pain—physical or emotional. This paradigm motivates all our decisions and is at the core of all our behavior. Fear of rejection or ridicule and our need for acceptance often lead us to strategies that prevent us from opening our hearts and being vulnerable, despite that being the path to deeper and more meaningful relationships. Choosing to escape into a device can feel safer than putting yourself out there, only to be dismissed or ignored. Hence there is a need to maintain awareness of your intention while making a change.

Making changes cannot be a passive process, as we are too wired to scout for danger and run away from anticipated pain. Furthermore, we tend to put our focus first on the kinds of thoughts and ideas to which our brain is trained to default. If you believe the world is a scary place, then you will default to looking for threats and danger. If, however, you believe the world is a safe place, then your brain will default to seeing people with loving kindness and trust. Instead of being passive (going unconsciously down our default brain pathways that, for many, lead to the world being a scary place), we need to be actively making different choices.

We can begin by identifying those moments when we gravitate towards avoidant behaviors. In those moments, it behooves us to take a pause and see how we can replace those old pathways with new ones that support connection and enhance pleasure. For example, the next time we find ourselves in an unfamiliar environment, rather than running home or immersing ourselves in our phone, we can take the opportunity to look up and make eye contact with, or even meet, at least one new person. We can start with something that might seem unthinkable: a warm, caring smile. Or, we can identify a situation we have felt uncomfortable addressing with a family member or friend and challenge ourselves to connect around it with vulnerability and authenticity. The opportunity here is to step out of our comfort zone and try something new. After all, has what you have been doing up until now really been working out? The connections may not always be as we hoped, but they consistently offer us occasions to learn, grow, and hone both our ability to connect and our sense of personal agency—key players in leading us out of the disconnection epidemic.

Our daughters have been blessed and cursed with opportunities to experience different schools. The positive has been building resilience, discovering unfamiliar and exciting teaching methods, and meeting new friends. The downside has been a lack of predictability and comfort and a loss of significant and dear friendships. With every move, we noticed an initial attachment to devices, virtual gaming, and favorite movies. The amount of time they desired to be on their devices proved to be more than we were comfortable with. Part of this was an effort to tether to the familiar. The other was the path of least resistance (avoiding pain over seeking pleasure). They could remain connected to what they know rather than step into the discomfort of the unknown. This was despite moving next door to two families with girls their same age. How easy it would be to step outside and meet the neighbors! Yet the avoidance of pain (possible rejection or discordance) trumped the potential for pleasure (making new friends). Change here was not happening naturally and needed active awareness and motivation. A family discussion around encouraging connection and discussing anything that might interfere with this need (such as extra device time) eventually drove our daughters next-door. What resulted were friendships that provide ongoing pleasure, fun, excitement, and joy. The take-home message is that work was initially required to replace default programming with new behaviors, yet the reward was well worth the effort.

Disconnection is a main cause of addiction

The focus of this book is not addiction, yet it is worth noting that connection is the key to overcoming addictive behaviors. When self-connection and connection to others are optimized, then addiction loses its power and value. Addiction (whether to food, work, alcohol, gambling, sex, or drugs) is not a disease that is inherited; rather, it is an attempt to escape pain—physical, mental, or emotional. This can be the pain of loss, physical pain as a result of illness or injury, loneliness, lack of social support, years of repression and suppression, trauma, all work and no play, and so on. To alleviate this pain, we medicate with our "drug" of choice (food, shopping, gambling, alcohol, or others). Yet the more you become aware of this pain inside of you and learn how to heal it instead of medicating it, the less you will continue to live in it as well as project it onto others. When you stop living in the pain, the "drugs" that you once employed to cope with it no longer provide any value.

Chapter 4

Why Doctors Are Teaching Connection

"We suffer not because we are in pain,
but because we are in pain alone."
—Dr. Naomi Ramen

Y OU MAY BE WONDERING why medical doctors would be spending time talking about connection. Isn't this an area for therapists? Or the last resort for patients who don't have any "real" medical issues?

Connection as we define it at WeHeal is your sense of participating in an authentic, caring relationship. This is usually with other people, but we expand that to include your relationship to yourself. As was discussed in Chapter 3, when you are not in an authentic, caring, and warm relationship with others, you experience a sense of disconnection and isolation. And as we now know, isolation has been shown to cause physical disease; in other words, isolation does not just present a problem for your spiritual and emotional well-being; it is actually a serious risk to your physical health.

An experiment demonstrating this phenomenon was conducted on monkeys, normally a social species, who were placed in isolation. Isolating the monkeys stimulated their fight-or-flight response, increasing "warrior" over "repair/restore" monocytes (a type of blood cell). The result was an increased state of inflammation in the body. In threat, the body revs up the production of warrior cells. When the body feels safe and there are no perceived threats, it sends signals to shift the balance from a preponderance of "warrior" monocytes to greater prevalence of "repair/restore" monocytes. This process is important to fight damaged cells, cancer, and other invaders as needed. In this isolation experiment, not only were more "warrior" cells produced but they also became insensitive to hormones that would normally dampen their inflammatory response. In addition, researchers found those white blood cells to be LESS effective in fighting off viruses and LESS effective at returning quickly back to health. Not surprisingly, when a second monkey was introduced, the "warrior" levels of the isolated monkey decreased and the sensitivity to fight infection and recovery increased. In other words, isolation isn't just a concern for stimulating feelings of depression; rather, isolation is a concern for stimulating powerful cellular changes in our body that affect our physical health, including inflammation and our body's ability to effectively fight cancer, viruses, and other invaders.[1]

At WeHeal, we see disconnection and the resulting isolation as multi-faceted. On one hand, we look at connection with other people. When you feel comfortable, safe, understood, and open with other people, you are going to experience a sense of connection. Our Essence of WeHeal (EoW) model helps enhance this connection by offering alternatives to the way we currently think about and communicate with others. Additionally, there is a connection to self. As a result of developmental trauma in childhood, many people have suppressed aspects of their authentic selves. For example, as a child, you may have enjoyed expressing care and affection by hugging, but your parents taught you that was "inappropriate." To maintain approval and connection with your parents, you learned to suppress the desire to hug. Over the years, you may have shifted from suppression (conscious avoidance) of your desire to hug people to repression (subconscious detachment), eventually identifying as "someone who doesn't like to hug" or who feels uncomfortable during an embrace. The cost of attachment to your parents, a survival necessity for a child, was to wall-off any "undesirable" parts of your authentic self.

The EoW model is aimed at identifying these areas of isolation and disconnection while restoring connection to our authentic selves. Interestingly, it takes energy and resources to maintain suppression and repression. Similarly, it takes effort to reconnect with yourself. This is especially so because your initial disconnection from yourself was for a good reason and served a purpose, primarily to gain acceptance, love, and connection with your caregivers (the people you deemed necessary for your survival). As a result, it may feel scary to release what has been bottled up for so long. You may even notice a strong resistance to doing so. This is where trust, knowledge, patience, and self-compassion come in: the trust that you are resilient and capable of handling what comes your way, the knowledge that you do not have to do this alone and that we are here to support you along your journey, and the patience to move at a pace that feels right to you and can be sustained over time. There is no benefit in pushing your limits to the point of overdoing it and giving up. And last, but not least, you will need to find the courage and compassion to reconnect to parts of yourself that for so long you have defined as "undesirable." Only through self-compassion can these parts of ourselves find the safety and space to awaken. If instead, they are met with judgment and criticism, the pain of opening up will be too great, and as a result, you will shut right down again.

The numerous studies on expressive writing help remind us of the health benefits we experience when we relieve our isolation by reconnecting to our authentic self. James Pennebaker did some of the pioneering work on expressive writing. What he discovered was profound; there was a significant physical impact from simply writing about traumatic or emotionally charged topics (compared to superficial events) for four consecutive days at 15-20 minutes a day. This included changes in brainwave patterns and skin conductance (a surrogate marker of our fight-or-flight response). Additionally, there were significant drops in blood pressure, heart rate, blood sugar, and frequency of doctor visits, among other health markers. Pennebaker and his colleagues also found improvements in immune system function, as well as physical health in general, including improved pain scores for people with fibromyalgia, irritable bowel syndrome, and various cancers.[2]

How could something so simple have such an impact on physical health? It is because there is such a huge cost to disconnecting and isolating parts of our authentic selves. By writing freely without censoring or restricting, we begin to release our innermost thoughts and feelings. Studies on expressive writing showed that simply releasing your suppressed thoughts onto a piece of paper was enough to begin to lessen the physiological damage and resulting chronic disease associated with isolating parts of your authentic self. Shredding the paper after we are finished writing, thus ensuring that no one will see it, adds an additional sense of safety to freely expressing ourselves.

A similar benefit is seen when we can connect with others. Studies have shown that when people who had been feeling disconnected and isolated were placed into small groups focused on empowerment, peer support, and enhanced social integration, they needed less healthcare support and lived longer.[3] Other research has found that diabetic patients who had highly empathic doctors had a significantly lower rate of serious complications compared to similar patients with low-empathy doctors. In other words, just by connecting with a doctor who understood and heard them, these patients did better.[4] Similarly, a study on 891 diabetic patients showed that those with physicians with high empathy scores (compared to physicians with low empathy scores) had 29% better blood sugar control (defined as hemoglobin A1c <7.0) as well as being 25% more likely to have a low level of "bad" LDL cholesterol (defined as < 100).[5] Trust, another important factor in connection, also plays a big role in the degree to which patients thrive. In a study in which patients received a painful stimulus, those who did not trust their doctor reported increased pain compared to those who did trust their doctor. In other words, patients' trust in their doctors has substantial impacts on pain.[6]

The evidence is irrefutable that isolation and disconnection cause real physical disease at the cellular, hormonal, and nervous system levels. It is clear that connection is not just an emotional nicety; rather, it is an essential part of optimizing physical health. We would be remiss to exclude it from our treatment paradigm. By spending time learning how to connect to your authentic self and to others more effectively while eliminating isolation, you begin to stimulate a sense of safety, health, and well-being where physical disease can reverse. Once we understood the mechanisms by which connection operates to influence our health, we knew that it was necessary to prioritize it at WeHeal.

CHAPTER 5

Our Model: Essence
of WeHeal

"It always seems impossible until it is done."
—NELSON MANDELA

BY NOW WE HAVE A BETTER understanding of why we don't feel great... why life is not yet wonderful.

- According to the CDC, one in three adults don't get enough sleep[1] and according to a poll conducted by YouGov, six in seven Americans wake up every single day of the week feeling tired and not refreshed.[2]
- We are regularly feeling emotions, yet half of these are negative or mixed in nature.[3]
- Looking at dietary guidelines from 2015-2020, over three-quarters of the population are not eating enough fruits and vegetables, while about two-thirds are over the limit for sugar and saturated fat consumption and 90% get too much sodium.[4]
- The U.S. Department of Health and Human Services reports that only one in three adults get enough physical activity each week and less than 5% engage in 30 minutes of physical activity daily.[5]
- A survey of 2000 adults found that one in four didn't have someone they could confide in, seven out of ten admitted holding back

true feelings when sharing with others, and nine in ten reported downplaying their emotions to avoid burdening a loved one.[6]

People often acknowledge that they have been burning the candle at both ends, feel exhausted and depleted, and are ultimately lonelier and more disconnected than ever. Yet they yearn for greater connection and enhanced joy and satisfaction in life. If happiness and joy are the currency they really value most, then how do they amass it? Despite common belief, it is not through the accumulation of wealth, status, and stuff. Yes, these things may be appealing and may introduce a certain comfort in our lives, but at best they result in temporary relief and fleeting pleasure rather than delivering true happiness and joy. After all, they are external validations rather than internal ones. No matter how much a person may have, unless they feel whole within, it is not enough.

On the other hand, meaning and purpose have been shown to enhance joy, satisfaction, and happiness. In a 2018 survey, nine out of ten people said they would trade money for a more meaningful job, even giving up 23% of their future earnings.[7]

Both in our personal and professional lives, the desire to feel whole is something that we have passionately sought out. It is what drives us to research, learn, and expand our skill set both personally and professionally. Over the years, we have amassed a wealth of information, and each time have added to our model for optimal health and well-being. It has never felt entirely complete until the creation of our Essence of WeHeal (EoW) model. The model is built around nine fundamental pillars of life. When fully optimized and in balance, these nine pillars will enable you to thrive beyond your expectations, taking you from wellness to wonderful. The pillars are centered around the self (you) and are comprised of your internal world—areas that you can enhance independently (sleep, nutrition, activity, and play)—and your external world—important relationships in your life, specifically family & friends, work, spirituality, and the natural world.

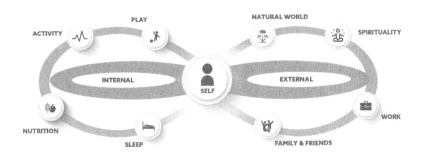

At the highest level, the EoW brings together three elements: Resourcing, Connection, and Regulation. Resourcing involves the optimization of our internal world and manifests as feeling energized, repleted, and resilient. It entails taking action to ensure that our body is getting the fuel and care it needs to function optimally. Connection relates to our most important relationships from self to others to the greater world. Forming the intention and acquiring the skills to deepen connection allows us to live our life with authenticity and compassion—enriching our experience and enhancing our joy. Regulation includes ideas and exercises for feeling safe and calm. Rewiring our brains to focus on messages of safety over default messages of danger plays a major role in regulation. This is achieved by noticing sensations, thoughts, and environmental factors through awareness and mindfulness. Mindfulness and awareness of your feelings deactivate the fear circuits in the brain as it learns these are not dangerous. This process disrupts the pain-fear cycle in the brain and helps you interpret signals more accurately and effectively.

The internal world of the EoW (Resourcing) starts with Self and consists of Nutrition, Activity, Play, and Sleep. We will include a high-level explanation of each of these and delve into them more deeply in further chapters. Self encourages us to discover, uncover, redefine, and compassionately connect to our inner being and authentic self. Nutrition identifies not only the foods we should eat for optimal health and well-being, but also our relationship to food and eating. Activity addresses the need for daily movement as well as the benefit of incorporating strength, cardio, flexibility, and balance into our routine. Play introduces the importance of content-free time that invites spontaneity, fun, and creativity with self and others without an agenda or need to be efficient and productive. Sleep is the quantity and quality of our rest. For most of us, eight hours is the ideal window of sleep time we need nightly. The sleep chapter will explore why we thrive on eight hours, what happens when we get less sleep, and how we can optimize our sleep hygiene.

The external world (Connection) of the EoW also centers on Self and highlights connection with Family and Friends, Work, Spirituality, and the Natural World. We will introduce the concept of connecting with the external world followed by a more in-depth explanation in later chapters. Connection centers on an authentic experience we have with ourselves and the world around us; it includes the goals we set for our lives. It creates meaning and purpose and gives us a sense of direction along our life's journey. This begins with the most important relationships in our lives: our family, friends, and work. Spirituality reminds us of our interdependence, that there is something that is bigger than us and that we are a part of it. And Natural World extends beyond humanity to animals, plants, and our environment.

Our hope with the EoW is to offer a continuum on which we can track our lives within a variety of categories that enhance health, well-being, and overall joy in how we experience ourselves and others. It is about flow and balance in the present moment, not a destination or goal to achieve. At any moment, any part of your life can be out of balance. The EoW provides a framework through which to evaluate where your attention needs to go to restore balance and flow.

Disease and pain are more likely to occur when flow is impaired or blocked. However, when your EoW is in a state of balance and flow, or you are even just heading in the direction of restoring balance and flow, then you will have significantly increased the chances for Life Is Wonderful in that moment. Each branch can be addressed separately, and we recommend people begin with the area that is most in need of attention and balance. However, in the same way that we desire and search to be whole, the real magic of the EoW is in the interwoven nature of its paradigm. For example, our level of regulation (how safe we feel and how far we are removed from fight-or-flight mentality) affects how much energy we can give to resourcing (in survival mode there is no time to optimize our internal world—sleep, nutrition, activity, and play). And how resourced we are impacts our ability to access and execute our connection skills. Similarly, the level of connection we experience in our life affects how safe and secure we feel (regulation) and again how much attention we can give to resourcing.

The EoW can thus be used as an internal barometer to gauge how close we are to a state of Life Is Wonderful in any given moment and from there identify where our attention can go. It serves as both an assessment tool for the present moment as well as a frame on which to direct future choices. Because some of the branches may be new and unfamiliar, the learning curve is exponential (begins slowly and rapidly grows) and continues to build on itself. So, while one may be overwhelmed at first, wondering where to start and what to focus on, over time it becomes a second nature body scan: where am I, what am I feeling, and where does my attention need to go?

In life, you need to head towards what you want, not avoid what you don't want. You can't get to Florida by trying not to go to New York. Connecting to your inner motivation will help you identify what you *do* want. Ask yourself, what is driving you? Why do you want to change? What do you want to learn and how do you want to grow? Once you are clear on this, create clear strategies that help you attain your goals. When we focus on what we don't want, we may indeed avoid unwanted things. But that is not the same as actually getting what we do want. For example, we can avoid eating chocolate cake but that won't necessarily help us lose weight, especially while we are still eating ice cream and cookies. If we really want quiet, we are unlikely to get it by simply asking our children to stop yelling. They may stop yelling and start banging drums.

Similarly, we need to practice noticing the feelings we DO enjoy, in order to increase the chances of experiencing them more often, bringing us closer to Life Is Wonderful. Unfortunately, most people tend to compartmentalize emotions in an effort to be in control and are therefore out of practice in noticing and naming their feelings. That is why taking time to stop, notice, and name our feelings is so important. And not just painful or unpleasant feelings, but also pleasant and joyful feelings (See Appendices D-F for support sheets). Try it now. For example, do you notice feeling jolly when playing with your kids or feeling light and expansive when watching the ocean? Can you feel the sun on your face, enjoy the embrace of someone you love, notice the experience of laughter? The more you practice noticing your feelings, the quicker you will be able to connect to what action was taken that resulted in that pleasant feeling and consider taking that same action again in the future. In other words, this practice helps you in the present moment while also increasing the chance of enjoying similar moments in the future!

Along your healing journey, remember that it is your inner motivation that determines long-term integration of new behaviors. If we want behaviors to last a lifetime, we cannot do things for external rewards or to avoid negative consequences. These extrinsic motivations are transient and cannot be relied on to always be there when you need them, whereas intrinsic motivation is always with you because it lives inside of you. By understanding why we want to do something for ourselves, we connect to our core values and needs. For example, we may be able to lose weight to look good for a family wedding. However, as long as the weight loss was just to look good for an event (extrinsic reward), once the event is over, we often gain back the weight. If instead, we connected our desire to lose weight to our value for health, then there is ongoing motivation to continue that behavior to remain true to our values.

Making changes can be stressful, especially if we are focused on getting it right. If we see every mistake as a stumbling block that is then received with self-judgment (blame, criticism, or shame, for example), the process becomes so uncomfortable or even painful that we inevitably give up. At the same time, judgments of self and others are automatic and thereby inescapable. This is especially so if you were brought up in a world where your parents, teachers, and supervisors used judgments to keep you "in line." Our brains are constantly monitoring how to keep us safe (and as an inherently social species, a large part of our safety relies on being accepted by our family and social circles). Reprimanding us harshly or scaring us when we make a mistake (as our parents, teachers, and supervisors often did) can be a familiar method for enforcing compliance with external values or rules; however, it is a tragic way to prevent undesired behaviors from happening again. What it teaches us are moralistic judgments that are then used to guide "right/wrong" behavior. Instead of trying to resist judgments that have become deeply habitual, we can make the counterintuitive choice to embrace them. Underneath judgments lie messages that we can choose how to interpret. Instead of taking them at face value, we can uncover what they are aiming to relay. Are they encouraging you to grow and change your behavior (for example wanting to ensure safety while driving by saying, "Are you crazy, driving while texting?") or trying to protect you from emotional pain (by saying, "Don't tell him you love him, you will only get hurt")? Regardless of the judgment, the opportunity we have is to take a beat and decipher the underlying message—in order to see what can be learned from it.

Remember, "mistakes" (merely doing something you wish you did differently, or not doing something you wish you did) are bound to happen; that is a valuable part of the learning process. If instead, we approach them with self-compassion and curiosity, understanding that we are going to "mess up" and taking the opportunity to grow and learn from these experiences, we are more likely to continue along that more joyful and satisfying path as well as reap much greater benefits from our efforts.

Learning from our default behaviors and getting clarity on where we want to head (as directed by our internal values, not external acceptance and approval) are two keys to optimizing our EoW. Awareness of these two keys allows us to better understand where we have come from and gives us greater compassion, as well as encouragement for where we are going. To truly benefit from the EoW, however, you must experience it. It cannot be intellectualized. Knowing how to eat healthy, what exercises to do, and how much sleep you need is not enough. In fact, optimization of your EoW is a lifelong adventure that continues to unfold as you go. For every person this will be a unique journey, tailored to the needs, goals, and dreams you have for your life. As you take your individual path, there are some important points to keep in mind.

1. Understand what comprises your internal and external worlds. Identify where you are most successful and what areas need attention. Start by focusing on your greatest needs. Note personal obstacles to optimization. The goal here is clarity: painting an accurate picture of where you are currently and where you want to go.

2. Prioritize the areas you believe will bring the greatest value. These are not necessarily the ones that need the most attention. The difference is subtle yet important. For example, you may have been completely sedentary to date, need to change your diet, and require more sleep. All of these areas need attention. However, your relationship with your partner, which has been tense lately, may be an area of greater value. Learning to communicate and connect to your partner can bring you greater companionship, enhanced intimacy, and more joy. The enriched partnership and resulting inspiration and hope can help you sleep better. Sleeping better can give you more energy to incorporate physical fitness. The more healthy habits you implement (sleep, activity, connection), the more likely you will be motivated to improve your life further (for example, by changing your diet).

3. Be curious and humble, not perfect. See mistakes not as failures but as opportunities to provide you with feedback. You can either succeed or learn but you cannot fail. Expect obstacles, as they are reflections of your efforts. The learning here is first to discern what worked for you and what did not. If you enjoyed the strategies that worked, by all means, continue them. For those that haven't worked, explore why not and how you might act differently knowing what you know now.

4. Don't give up. Perseverance is key. The reality is that we all veer off our paths occasionally—it's practically inevitable. So, rather than focus on trying to prevent derailments, learn how to identify them as well as how to get back on your path. The earlier

you can recognize a digression, the easier it will be to re-focus your efforts and get back to where you want to be.

5. Measure your progress not as the absence of unwanted behaviors, but as a decrease in frequency, magnitude, and duration of unwanted behaviors over time. In that way, you will experience more joy and satisfaction around your personal growth.

CHAPTER 6

A New Perspective on Chronic Disease

"The most important decision we make is whether we
believe we live in a friendly or hostile universe."
—ALBERT EINSTEIN

B EFORE WE JUMP INTO the "solution," it is essential that people understand the role of inflammation in the body. These days, inflammation is a buzzword associated with illness and disease, and much of
the wellness industry has become focused on combating inflammation.
In this effort, there is a kernel of truth mixed into a lot of noise and confusion. Inflammation is actually a necessary reaction to repair damage
in our physical body. It is a response to threats such as cuts, infections,
or broken bones. This threat response activates the immune system to
mount an inflammatory cascade, sending a variety of resources, including red and white blood cells, to "clean" and repair tissue in the
body. Ideally, it is turned on when we need repair and turned off once
the tissue is healed. Polyvagal theory, developed by Stephen Porges,
Ph.D., helps us understand how our body responds to perceived threat
or danger, and the effects of those two distinct physiological states on
our overall health.

Living in a constant state of threat or high alert upsets this essential
system. Instead of healing true tissue damage (the actual "tiger"), the
inflammatory response is triggered by non-tissue threats (perceiving

or imagining that the "tiger" is there or will be coming soon). Since there is no tissue to heal in these situations, the inflammatory response gets "confused" and is unable to appropriately shut off. As a result, we develop chronic inflammation that over time leads to illness and disease.

Polyvagal theory helps us make sense of how this works, specifically when it comes to activating our immune system's inflammatory response to non-tissue threats. What is important to remember is that, whether it is a real threat or a perceived threat, our body responds in the same way. The difference is that with a real threat, the inflammatory cascade fixes what it needs to and then allows the tissues to heal. In a perceived threat, all of the compounds are still released in the inflammatory cascade, but since there is no physical tissue damage to fix, they linger around, building up a state of chronic inflammation.

Polyvagal theory explains how many different organs in the body are connected by the large vagus nerve (a cranial nerve starting in the brain and affecting many organs, including the heart, lungs, stomach, and intestines) and are affected by how we feel as well as our perception of the world around us. The vagus nerve and the various nuclei within it support two different physiological states in our body: the state of safety and the state of danger or threat. When in the physiological state of threat or high alert, we become hypervigilant and prepare all systems to fight the perceived danger. This cascade of changes happens in the body to increase the chances that we will survive whatever we believe is threatening us. For example, we halt cellular "housekeeping" activities (such as those removing mutated cells that can turn into cancer) to shift resources towards threat neutralization, our heart beats faster (to pump more blood wherever fuel is most needed), we shunt blood towards our extremities (to power our arms to fight and legs to flee) and hindbrain (to defend by reacting immediately, as opposed to thinking and analyzing), our cells secrete proinflammatory cytokines (to prepare for tissue damage in response to the threat), we secrete adrenaline, cortisol, and histamine into our bloodstream (to further support the body to be able to fight or flee), and there are even changes in the muscles in our body such as the middle ear (to better hear certain sounds consistent with threat or harm) and muscles in our larynx (so that our voices can signal threat to others). These are just a few of the many changes our body undergoes to prepare to fight the tiger, bear, or whatever it believes is threatening our life. The threat response lives within us as a subconscious survival mechanism. We can't turn it on at will, nor can we turn it off at will.

It is important to note that our body reacts to a perceived threat as it does to a real threat. Much of what we perceive as threat is shaped by our upbringing, specifically how our caregivers treated us, how they saw the world, and what they taught us to be afraid of. A child brought up in an environment where care was consistent, their experiences were acknowledged, and their needs supported, tend to perceive people and the world around them very differently than a child who was physically abused, emotionally neglected, and experienced many unmet needs.

So how does this system work? We often hear people talk about our sympathetic nervous system (which mediates our survival response), or the fight-or-flight response. These are essentially the same thing: our body trying to protect us from danger. We have two survival states to deal with danger. Our more preferred, or more developed, state to fight off danger is to mobilize and fight or flee. This must be done in short bursts because, after a period of time, we will run out of energy to remain mobilized. The other state, which can happen when we see that mobilization is not working or we are facing imminent death, is immobilization. This freeze/faint response is a more primitive state of defense and is our body's last attempt to save resources or, at the very least, dissociate if we are about to be killed. This immobilization state is frequently experienced by trauma victims who will say that they can't remember what happened or they did nothing to defend themselves. This was not because they were weak or didn't care; rather, it was because their nervous system put them into a defensive posture of immobilization in a last-ditch effort to try to help them survive.

What most people don't realize is that our baseline state is mobilization. This differs from a more common, yet erroneous, thought that our baseline is a state of calm and we mobilize when we feel threatened. The reality is that being in a constant state of mobilization is a survival advantage. This allows us to always be ready to fight or flee from a threat. We are wired to assume danger until safety is established. Otherwise, the seconds it might take to activate fight-or-flight could mean the difference between life and death. Imagine seeing the tiger coming toward you. It is not hard to understand the advantage of just running versus having to shift from calm to preparing to run.

To leave our baseline mobilized state, we need to actively turn on a sense of safety. What is our "safety brake?" How do we slow down or tell our baseline mobilized nervous system to calm down and take a break? Through perceived messages of safety experienced in our environment. This process is called neuroception, a term coined by Dr. Porges to emphasize that our nervous system must actually experience the perception. We cannot just think we are safe; instead, we must give our body the felt sense that it is safe (as accurately perceiving whether one is safe or in danger could be a matter of life or death, it is too important to trust our thoughts alone).

It is in this state of safety that our body shifts our physiology from supporting fighting, fleeing, freezing, or fainting (types of threat responses to perceived danger) to supporting the processes of resting, digesting, healing, and reproducing (all of which can happen only when we are in a state of perceived safety). Organs involved in resting, digestion, healing, and reproduction require a steady stream of "you are safe" messaging (flowing through our vagus nerve as part of our autonomic nervous system) to be able to optimally function. For example, your gastrointestinal system requires a steady stream of "you are safe" messaging for the gut to function normally. In threat mode, safety messages are shut off to optimize our chances of survival. Resources shift from the gut to our extremities, heart, and lungs. These are the areas that will help us fight harder or flee faster. As such, most people with chronic gut-related issues, for example, will not only benefit from significant dietary intervention but will also often have an excessive level of chronic mobilization compounding the picture.

Sadly, in this day and age, so many of us live in a chronic state of threat or high alert that we really struggle to apply our safety brake. Most people don't even realize that they are chronically mobilized. This often happens because threats are no longer just physical threats (the snake, bear, or tiger in front of you) but also mental threats (worries about keeping a job or paying bills), emotional threats (worries about disconnection from family and friends), and spiritual threats (senses of isolation or lack of purpose and meaning in life). Unlike physical threats, mental, emotional, and spiritual threats follow us around because we can't run from them like we can a snake or bear. To cope, we turn to food, alcohol, gambling, shopping, cigarettes, and drugs—anything we can find to dull or numb the pain and discomfort. Unfortunately, these tragic strategies are further perceived by our body as dangerous, thereby continuing to trigger the inflammatory response working to protect us and neutralize the threat.

In survival mode, there are many ways we interrupt messages of safety. The result is a chronically activated, mobilized—or worse, immobilized—defensive state. We do this through our actions, specifically through the things we say, think, and do. What we *say*, how we *think*, and what we *do* are mostly determined by our society and the culture in which we grew up. Many of us grew up in or currently live in a society and culture that normalizes toxic communication, thoughts, and behavior, all of which trigger a sense of threat. How we learn to respond to common stressors such as unpredictability, lack of information, insecurity, and conflict determines whether we enter into a threat response or safety response. For many of us, the default is sensing threat; therefore, the healing that needs to take place is a shift to communicating, thinking, and behaving in a manner that stimulates a sense of safety. For example, we can help deliver messages of safety by connecting with our choice in everything we do versus convincing ourselves we are victims of our life's circumstances. In essence, we are empowered (safe) versus helpless (in danger). If I succumb to a state of being overwhelmed or hopeless because I am feeling stressed with all that I have to do, I become a victim of my hectic and demanding life. As a result of thinking this way, I will enter into a threat response that stimulates the proinflammatory cascade and defensive posture of either fight, flee, or freeze. On the other hand, framing the same stress from a perspective of choice gives me a sense of encouragement and agency.

In this mind frame, I see that I am feeling overwhelmed because I have chosen to schedule myself in such a way that I don't have enough breaks or opportunities for self-care. As a result, I lack the sense of comfort and inner peace I desire, and instead feel pressured and stressed. Notice how I still may choose to work while feeling overwhelmed, but by simply reframing it as my choice, I promote feelings of empowerment and agency that support a sense of safety instead of threat.

People who have experienced a lot of Adverse Childhood Experiences (or ACEs) will likely have nervous systems that have been "tuned" and geared up to prepare for threat. Because they have spent more time in threat mode, their safety brake system is less developed and slower to respond. In essence, like any other unused muscle, it has atrophied to some extent. As adults, it may be harder for them to apply the brake. If you grow up believing the world is a dangerous place, is it any wonder you are not as willing to believe, trust, or know how to receive messages of safety? People living in a baseline state of threat or high alert tend to be more easily activated and reactive, and suffer more chronic disease (remember, the state of threat or high alert is a proinflammatory state ready to fight and prepare for damage control in the body.) According to the CDC, "ACEs are linked to chronic health problems, mental illness, and substance misuse in adulthood. Furthermore, preventing ACEs can help children and adults thrive and potentially lower the risk for conditions like depression, asthma, cancer, and diabetes in adulthood."[1]

Chronic pain is another area affected by this threat vs. safety system. Interestingly, chronic pain ranks as one of the most pervasive and troubling issues in our Western health system. This is not only expensive but also debilitating. According to the CDC, one in five adults and nearly one in three people over 65 live consistently with chronic pain.[2] At the same time, we have very little to offer in the way of medications and procedures to effectively treat chronic pain. That is because, for many people, the issue is neural pathway pain that occurs when we are in a state of threat or high alert.

Most people don't know that pain is actually generated in the brain when it perceives damage or danger of damage in the body. For example, when you break a bone or cut your skin, the brain will generate pain sensations to protect the damaged area so that it doesn't move or get damaged further, thereby allowing the tissue to heal. In this scenario, the brain generates pain signals in response to a real threat, the threat of moving a damaged or hurt body part before it fully heals. This is a wonderful system for acute pain. Without it, people would die. In fact, not being able to feel pain is a serious disorder; people afflicted by it often don't live past their twenties.[3]

When we are in a state of chronic perceived threat, however, the brain continues to help us however it can. It stimulates pain sensations down old neural pathways, even though it is addressing threats not from actual tissue damage but rather all the non-tissue threats we discussed above. This vigilance occurs because the brain cannot distinguish between physical, mental, emotional, and spiritual threats. They are treated equally as threats and as such the body responds consistently to try to protect us. In a state of chronic threat, the brain tries to help warn us and keep us safe, including signaling pain despite the absence of tissue damage. Over time, this becomes chronic pain in response to non-tissue threats. The presence of chronic pain incites anxiety and worry, compounding the problem by further signaling threat. So instead of the threat being resolved after six weeks of healing of bone or tissue, we have this compounding emotional, mental, and/or spiritual threat that could, if not appropriately addressed, last months, years, or a lifetime. It is hard for people to really comprehend that mental and physical pain can generate the same physiological response, but it is essential to do so if they want to heal the chronic pain arising from non-tissue threats.

A groundbreaking study demonstrated the impact of Pain Reprocessing Therapy (PRT), a therapy designed to specifically target neural pathway pain. Participants suffering chronic pain for an average of about nine years were randomized to PRT which included participating in one telehealth session with a physician and in eight psychological treatment sessions over four weeks. Treatment was primarily aimed to help patients reconceptualize their pain as due to non-dangerous brain activity rather than peripheral tissue injury, using a combination of cognitive, somatic, and exposure-based techniques. The results were impressive! Two-thirds of the participants (who had chronic pain for an average of nine years prior) randomized to PRT were pain-free or nearly pain-free at post-treatment (reporting a pain intensity score of 0 or 1 out of 10) and sustained it at the twelve-month follow-up. What's more, the impact of PRT was more than three times as effective as the placebo and more than six times as effective as usual conventional care![4]

Matt's story and the Essence of WeHeal

I was personally impacted by this healing paradigm. I experienced 9 months of intense, unrelenting lower back pain and sciatica that started after a particularly challenging turn of events in my life, despite following a nearly "perfect" diet, exercise, and sleep routine. My chronic pain was so bad that I was considering surgery, although surgery had never been shown to effectively treat low back pain. Unfortunately, people, including myself, are willing to do nearly anything (like pursue surgery that has no data supporting it) when desperate. This experience prompted a deeper exploration for a much more comprehensive approach to healing, out of which came the nine pillars of the Essence of WeHeal (Chapter 5). Implementing each of the pillars, some of which include aspects of PRT, was what ultimately gave me the results I was looking for. I have been sciatica-free ever since, without any surgery, pain medication, or other invasive interventions. The great news is that the support the Essence of WeHeal provides clients will not only address the causes of neural pathway pain in any body part, but it will also address additional areas in life that are erroneously triggering the threat defense system. As such, clients improve many areas of their health, in addition to their chronic pain.

How are we able to heal things that happened to us as far back as early childhood? Gabor Mate, MD, a trauma expert, likes to say that what matters is not what happened to you; rather what matters is what happened inside of you because of what happened to you. Much of what you do today, what you eat, the language you speak, is not a conscious choice; rather, it is simply the result of how we were brought up. However, we can choose to eat differently or speak different languages if we want. Similarly, how we react to our environment—what we say, think, and do—is often just a result of how we were brought up. However, we can consciously choose to say, think, and do things differently if we are so inclined. In other words, you do not have to be a victim of what happened to you in the past; you can change as soon as you are aware and ready.

Someone once said, "Resentment is like cutting your arm and waiting for the other person to die." There is a difference between being a victim and blaming others versus taking responsibility for the changes you wish to make. Our goal is to shift out of the toxicity of resentment and blame for what happened in the past and make room for greater agency in growing into the person you want to be today. Other people are still responsible for what they did to you, but only you are responsible for what you are going to do now and in the future. We like to think of your autonomic nervous system as a guitar string that can be tuned too tight; similarly, your threat awareness and prevention system can be tuned to be biased towards perceiving threat (often due to how we were raised as children). The good news, again, is that the WeHeal EoW can help you re-tune your nervous system towards a sense of safety by "working out" your safety brake "muscles." Like any other muscles in your body, you can choose to work them out, allowing them to grow and strengthen over time. Cultivating new behaviors (around the things we say, think, and do) geared towards supporting a sense of safety is just the workout your nervous system needs. Fortunately, this workout happens to be a fundamental feature of the EoW.

Humans are designed to be social, connected animals that thrive when connected to others. Humans will not thrive in disconnection and isolation. Disconnection and isolation are highly "dangerous" experiences for humans. In other words, connection is one of the main ways to trigger a sense of safety in our bodies and shut off the proinflammatory threat response. When people say things (communicate) in a way that meets needs for respect, warmth, and care (instead of raging, shaming, or guilting), then we stimulate a sense of safety in ourselves and others. When people think in a way that allows them to honor their internal feelings and needs (instead of suppressing and repressing their authentic selves) or they think in a way that helps them identify other people's underlying needs (instead of blaming and judging others), then they stimulate a sense of safety. When people think in ways that demonstrate compassion for the old belief systems they developed as children or young adults (trying to make sense of their world and stay attached to their "caregivers") but then transform them into new beliefs empowering them to honor their values, then they stimulate a sense of safety. When people do things such as showing compassionate and caring facial movements (ex: smiling), talking to us with a certain tone of voice, moving in a way that feels calm and peaceful, or holding space to "be" instead of "do," they stimulate a sense of safety. And when people do things (behaviors) such as sleep, eat, drink, move, and play in ways that are health-promoting and not toxic, then the body experiences a sense of safety.

The beauty of our nervous system is that it works in a bidirectional fashion. In other words, we can feel safe inside and as a result be open to connecting with others, or we can connect with others and then, as a result of that connection, start to feel safe inside. Connection helps us feel safe, and feeling safe helps us connect. We can feel happy and, as a result, smile—or we can smile and actually start to feel happy inside as a result. If you want to experience Life Is Wonderful, then say, think, and do things to help those around you perceive safety. By optimizing your EoW you will be doing just that. We will help you learn how to "stack your deck" towards safety so that your nervous system can easily and effectively apply your "safety brake," and effortlessly enter into a pro-social, anti-inflammatory state that supports your ability to not only rest, digest, heal, and reproduce, but also experience joy, satisfaction, and a state of Life Is Wonderful.

For additional information and key points, see Appendix C—"Physiological States and Nine Pillars of the Essence of WeHeal."

CHAPTER 7

Self

Pillar 1

"We are so accustomed to disguise ourselves to others
that in the end, we become disguised to ourselves."
—FRANCOS DE LA ROCHEFOUCAULD

To do what you truly want, you need an awareness of what is
going on inside of you. It is for this reason that the first area we
look at with people's EoW is the Self. When we are disconnected from
the sensations inside of us, we cannot feel fully alive or experience Life
is Wonderful. Self-care, or caring for oneself, is essential to thriving, and
yet sadly we are not doing enough of it. Unfortunately, many people
believe that self-care is only possible if we have enough time and/or
enough money. And if our self-care finally makes it onto our schedule,
it is the first to go when other needs arise. We are great at protecting
agreements and plans with other people, but we are lousy at protecting
similar agreements and plans with ourselves. Because so many of us live
in survival mode, in a state of scarcity with not enough time and not
enough money, self-care is a luxury we often feel we cannot indulge in.

Unlike self-improvement, which is about working harder and
smarter to fix defects and faults, thereby making us "better," self-care is
about loving and caring for ourselves moment to moment. It is about
connecting to our true selves and coming from that place of authenticity. Reframing the term in this manner makes it easy to see that the
only thing we need is an intention to care for ourselves in the present.
Self-care does not need to be lavish or lengthy; instead, it could mean

a two-minute breathing break when you start feeling tense; it could mean playing your favorite music on your drive home. It might mean choosing a healthier option for lunch over a less healthy one or recognizing you would enjoy a walk over a run. Maybe it will mean hibernating in bed rather than socializing with friends or choosing to read a book rather than watching a movie. Ultimately, self-care is a connection to yourself that allows you to reach inwards and discover what you like and what you don't, what resonates with your values and what does not, what brings you to life and what withers your soul.

Self-connection rewards you, allowing you to be honest with what lies inside your heart. To be able to discern what your soul truly desires is essential for thriving because even if you choose not to meet your needs in the moment, naming them honors their existence and makes it clear that they matter. When we connect to that inner authenticity we experience vulnerability, we learn about ourselves—what we enjoy and what we do out of obligation, where we are and where we want to go, and what we want to hold on to and what we are ready to release. In this state, we have an opportunity to discover things we have buried deep (suppressed and repressed) and learn how to heal by facing them. We can develop the skills to empathize, find acceptance, and even let go. Ultimately this authentic flow of our own life energy provides us with a sense of inner peace, security, and harmony.

Sadly, in a world where we continue to push forward by burning the candle at both ends, prioritizing self-connection is harder than it sounds. Chronic under-resourcing (not having enough resources such as food, water, or rest) creates stress. And lingering stress is associated with many health issues, including increased inflammation, heart disease, anxiety, depression, obesity, eating disorders, gastrointestinal issues (reflux, gastritis, ulcerative colitis, and irritable bowel syndrome), impaired immune function, and decreased resilience and overall ability to cope.

The perception of threat leading to stress is easily triggered in this survival mode state. Our brain, to protect us and keep us safe, runs an ongoing check of our surroundings to discern what is dangerous and what is not. This proved essential to our survival evolutionarily. We needed to see the saber-toothed tiger well in advance of it approaching us. As a result, our brain scan often happens subconsciously and trumps our conscious efforts to think otherwise.

When we go into a stress response, we shut off certain parts of our brain. Specifically, we shut off those areas of our brain responsible for executive functioning and regulating our emotions. The result is a decreased ability to connect with others, difficulty making decisions, loss of empathy, diminished capacity for ethical and moral judgments, and a lack of remorse. In addition, we lose our ability to reason, have insight, or make rational decisions. Simultaneously, paranoia, misperceptions, and prejudice increase as our bias tips toward the world, and the people in it, being dangerous. We begin to see ongoing and daily messages of danger. We may work long hours with no breaks and at times need to multitask to get it all done (which in turn maintains a sense of danger, in this case, a fear of dropping one of the many balls we are juggling). We tend to act out of obligation because we believe it's the right thing to do or are afraid to say "no." We live in artificial harmony where we suppress or repress our feelings and needs, ultimately sacrificing our true selves in order to fit in and get along or be a "good" parent, husband, student, or child. We experience environmental stressors including social media, news, traffic, pollution, noise, poverty, and discrimination. Some of these signals of danger can be physical threats such as injury, infections, and even sounds, bright lights, bad tastes or smells. Others, which can be just as triggering, come in the form of emotional pain, such as verbal abuse, abandonment, neglect, disapproval, criticism, social isolation, teasing, bullying, and excommunication. Regardless of the stimuli, the final effect is the same: we perceive a threat, which results in stress that over time becomes chronic and is ultimately dangerous for our health and well-being.

So, what can we do?

We must begin by addressing and tending to any states of stress. Stress is a normal part of life; however, evolutionarily, stress was sporadic and finite. We saw the tiger, we ran from the tiger, and we made it to safety. That was the winning formula. Our environment today challenges our ability to let go of stressors because they are ever-present. And beyond the physical, we now have the psychological. We no longer need to see the "tiger." We just need to *believe* the "tiger" (boss, bills, problems with kids) is coming or at least *worry* that the "tiger" will come. That perception alone ignites the stress response. The problem is that this perception has no end. We continue to believe the "tiger" is coming and, as long as we do, we remain in that stress response. The result is lingering chronic stress and its associated complications for our health and well-being.

Our youngest daughter, Jordan (age 8), had just experienced bullying at school with some older kids that stimulated fear, embarrassment, and discomfort. The situation was so distressing that it led to tears and her getting picked up early that day. So many needs went unmet in this instance, among them security, comfort, agency, and empowerment. We began the healing process with some empathy for her experience. This was followed by role-playing aimed to empower her with some responses she could use should she encounter those kids again. Jordan was feeling encouraged and ready to head back to school.

The next morning at drop-off, she saw the same children and responded by ducking under her window and asking to go home. It was two minutes to eight and I had an eight o'clock call I needed to take. I felt torn. I wanted to support my daughter and help in her time of need. I was also sad that she was feeling scared, and anxious to make my call. Normally I might have encouraged Jordan to find her courage and remember what we discussed the night before. However, in this moment, I realized that would most likely result in her pushing through as she suppressed her true feelings. Instead, I asked her empathically if she was feeling tightness in her belly, nervous, or even scared and worried there was danger ahead. She immediately resonated with that. I then explained this was her body and brain trying to protect her and asked her if we could discuss some options she had. She could stay in the car with me until I was done with my call, she could go straight to her classroom and let her teacher know what was happening, she could stay with her sister this morning or find a friend she trusted and hang out with them, or she could suggest another strategy to both navigate and honor her danger signals being stimulated. Although getting empathy and having options didn't make the situation go away, it did give Jordan a newfound sense of empowerment. Going from brain to heart gave her the messages of safety she needed to feel comfortable about going into the school.

She got out of the car. Heading into the yard, she planned what she would say to the kids in case they approached her. Before stepping in, she turned to me and gave me a thumbs up—letting me know she was okay. All the same, after taking my call in the parking lot, I checked up on her afterwards. She shared that the support and care she received helped her keep calm and remain comfortable and confident. This experience taught her body that she could resolve her own dilemma and face her fears while being supported by others who cared about her.

Acknowledging our stress raises our awareness and allows us to gain clarity. Once we know what feels dangerous, we can give it our attention. Giving something our attention does not equate to making it go away, understanding it, or fixing it. Instead, it gives us the opportunity to have compassion for ourselves and our experiences. When we can connect to ourselves or others (Jordan in the above example) with empathy and compassion, we get out of our heads and into our hearts. Unlike our brain which is constantly scanning for danger, our hearts seek to regulate, soothe, care for, and love us. From this space of loving care, we generate messages of safety. This starts with the comfort that we can show up as we are and feel as we do. Not having to repress, suppress, pretend, be something we are not, or feel things we simply don't, helps us experience peace of mind—the ultimate sense of safety and security.

Unfortunately, showing up authentically is an uphill battle and can be extremely difficult. As infants and children, we rely on our parents' care. Authenticity takes a back seat to survival. As a result, we prioritize pleasing our parents even when that means suppressing our true selves. If our parents don't support our unpleasant emotions, over time we learn to suppress rather than share them. We buy into statements such as "get over it," "turn that frown upside down," or "you think you have it bad, look at the kids in…" The fear that motivates this suppression of self is a fear we will not survive, be accepted, be loved, or be safe and secure if we show our true colors. We eventually identify with the suppressed reality and over time begin to believe that to be our true nature.

However, suppression comes at a great cost. Hiding our true self is a message of danger—it is too perilous to show who we really are so we must keep it buried: suppressed (conscious) or repressed (unconscious). This fuels a fight-or-flight response that results in a mobilized state in which we are ready to act as needed to survive. As we have discussed, regularly being in this state of stress produces a whole host of negative, proinflammatory impacts on our health and well-being.

Additionally, the loss of connection to our own heart—to what is alive and true for us, to our authenticity—is a form of trauma. Remember, if trauma is what happens inside of you because of what happens to you, then the changes in our bodies and our bodies' reactions occur not as a result of the trauma itself, but rather from our perception and experience of the traumatic event. If the brain embeds a situation as terrifying and dangerous, it will compartmentalize that awful, scary experience. In essence, it cuts us off from feeling the pain. As a result, many people who have experienced trauma feel a certain numbness, dissociation, or disconnection. Sadly, when we cut ourselves off from feeling unpleasant emotions, we also cut ourselves off from feeling pleasant emotions. Unless we learn to reactivate our connection to our body, to feel both pleasant and unpleasant emotions, and to trust that we can (especially with the right support system) process and heal, we will struggle to truly thrive in a state of Life is Wonderful. The good news is that although we cannot change what happened to us, with the right support and self-care, we can change what happens inside of us as a result of what happened to us.

In discussing trauma, we want to make clear our desire to empower and provide hope. We do not minimize the impact of trauma (big or small), and we understand the various degrees to which trauma can be experienced in different people's lives. It is for this reason that the

WeHeal team includes a variety of options to support the path to trauma recovery.

Practicing self-empathy is one strategy to bring us out of our heads and into our hearts, thus helping us connect to our authentic self. The key to self-empathy is to connect to the underlying feelings and unmet needs you have in the present. It's about empathizing with yourself the way you would empathize with someone else, by accompanying them on their experience in the moment. Here is an example of Wendy voicing "self-empathy," speaking aloud to herself, after an argument with her husband, Jim.

"Oh, Wendy, are you feeling angry and hurt? Do you really wish your conversation with Jim was more connected?" (She takes a deep breath and sighs, actions which are ways to self-regulate and calm her nervous system.) "Hmmm yes, how nice it would feel to just slow things down so that you could come from, and be received from, a place of kindness and compassion. When you think of how angry Jim was, seeing his face and hearing the tone of his voice, do you notice your body contracting? Yes, there's the contraction. And do you feel your shoulders tense and your throat tighten? Are you noticing an unsettled sensation in your gut that may feel uncomfortable?" (She breathes more breaths as she spends time with herself.) "Breathing into that state, what else do you feel, Wendy? Maybe some sadness or hurt? Those feelings are all welcome and we can just be with them without trying to stop them, change them, fix them, or hurry them. We don't have to get into the story of what happened, who is to blame, or what we need to do in the future. Wendy, I am here with you and your feelings as you allow them to flow through. And I am getting just how much you long to be able to have disagreements with Jim while still being warm, gentle, and connected with each other. I can sense just how painful it is for you to feel this disconnection right now and you are not alone."

As you can see, self-empathy connects to what is alive in yourself at the moment. In this case, it was a need for mourning, wishing for more connection. Furthermore, self-empathy is about being with and allowing your experience, not trying to suppress it or rectify it. Remember, as you practice, to let go of trying to fix it, defend it, blame others, sympathize, reassure, understand, or react. Instead, be open to feeling your truth, whatever that is, even if it is unpleasant. It is this connection that begins the healing process.

Feelings catcher

Our daughter likes to use a "feelings catcher" (similar to a dream catcher) where she imagines that her feelings flow from her heart and then out through her body and into the "feelings catcher" bracelet around her wrist. From there, her feelings flow out of her hand, transforming into bubbles that float into the universe. This exercise provides a sense of acceptance of feelings, an essential step for integration and processing. She describes the experience in her body using color, texture, temperature, flavor, sensation, movement, images, feelings, and needs. For example, when she connects to her sadness, she might describe a cold, dark blue, smooth, sour heaviness that sinks into her chest and travels to her throat. She then is able to track this more "tangible" form of her sadness as it flows from her chest and throat. When it is ready, the sadness might move down her arm, out to her "feelings catcher," and then into the air as bubbles. As she is doing this she will (by herself, or sometimes with a little help) also connect her sadness to her need for more care or love or whatever underlying need is triggering the feelings.

Allowing feelings to manifest and giving them "substance" supports their flow through our bodies. The acceptance and support of this natural flow are what allows life to flow. In fact, move-

ment, energy, and flow are what differentiate the body from being alive versus dead.

Doing this may seem like work at first, but, like everything else we do, it gets easier over time. Don't let your natural desire to conserve energy and avoid extra work dissuade you. When you don't support your feelings by being present and allowing them to flow, you impair your ability to experience the inner peace necessary to experience Life Is Wonderful.

Matt's story—expressing feelings

Over the years, I've learned to try to notice what I am feeling sooner, especially when it comes to anger. My wife and children have encouraged me by sharing that they actually feel more comfortable when I share my anger than when I try to suppress it, despite looking angry. My wife has learned to say things like, "It's okay that you are angry, and I just want to let you know that you don't have to be alone with your anger." My kids have learned to say, "Dad, you seem a little tense, is there anything you would like to do to support that tension?" And I have learned to say to myself, "Hello anger my friend, you are welcome to be here. What important needs of mine are you trying to bring my attention to?" Of course, you can find the language that resonates with you, but the key here is that my anger is not just about me; it affects everyone in the family. Therefore, everyone is working together to support the presence and acceptance of my feelings in a way that works for all of us. I sometimes follow my daughter's example and use the "Feelings Catcher" to make my anger more tangible. By doing this I am able to stop the suffering that results from resisting the emotion and instead support the flow and integration of my feelings, which stimulates inner peace and ultimately a state of Life Is Wonderful.

It is so important to remember that this works for both pleasant and unpleasant feelings. Both are just life happening. Allowing that life to "happen" is what brings us peace and satisfaction in our lives. Allowing all unpleasant feelings to flow allows us to feel a sense of peace and calm, whereas resisting their flow results in suffering as they remain with you longer than they or you want them to. Feelings are by definition transient; they can come and go by the minute. That is the beauty of feelings: they are connected to the present. When we worry about holding onto feelings we want or resisting feelings we don't want, that is when the suffering begins.

The transience of feelings, however, is dependent on us not suppressing or repressing them. Don't believe me? Try being happy... forever. Or sad... forever. Clearly, it doesn't work that way. Feelings come and go by the minute and are often stimulated by our thoughts, which can stick around. Further, staying aware of your feelings through an experience prevents the limiting beliefs that arise from suppression and repression. When we are afraid of feeling sadness or anger or fear, we avoid the situations in which they may arise. We limit our experience, and the world around us becomes small and constricted. This also sends our brain the message that these feelings are dangerous, triggering our threat response. Allowing ourselves to feel and trusting we can handle our emotions expands our opportunities to experience life with all of its ups and downs. This empowerment brings with it resilience, safety, and security.

Proficiency in self-empathy takes practice, time, and patience. As you work on developing that skill, some additional strategies for shifting to messages of safety include:

1) Expressive writing: In this exercise, the goal is to write whatever comes to mind without censoring, analyzing, or proofreading. Once you have completed your writing, you may cut, shred, or rip it up. The act of releasing repressed and suppressed emotions lowers the fight-or-flight stress response. It also helps raise awareness, while simultaneously creating some separation between our thoughts and our feelings. In addition, it identifies and acknowl-

edges pleasant as well as unpleasant emotions. Acknowledging our feelings is what allows them to integrate and dissolve naturally. Our brain, ever scanning for danger, otherwise tips the scale towards remembering unpleasant emotions that keep us feeling unsafe, continuing old behaviors meant to protect us, and raising our anxiety.

2) Cognitive soothing and somatic tracking: Sensations in our body, similar to feelings, may elicit worry or unpleasant emotions. As such, we may try to make sense of them, fix them, or suppress and repress them. Any of these strategies helps solidify a sense of danger. Instead, we can lean into these sensations, noticing them without necessarily reacting to them. In most cases, we may be surprised. Sensations are finite; they come and go. What empowers them and allows them to linger is our own continued attention to them. Scratching an itch often aggravates it rather than relieving it. If instead we sit back and notice the itch, accept the discomfort, and just observe, it eventually goes away. Try it yourself. The next time you notice an itch, instead of scratching it, notice how long you have to wait for the itch to naturally go away. The time will vary in different situations, depending on how mobilized and under-resourced you are. In addition, if you have thoughts that this itch will never end and feel panicked, then you will have a much longer wait than if you self-soothe and remind yourself this is just an itch and there is no reason to be afraid of it, as it will go away soon. This same process works for most of the other sensations we feel in our body, too!

3) Self-regulation: It takes about twenty minutes to extinguish the adrenaline rush that comes with a fight-or-flight stress response.[1] During that time, we can actively participate in regulation practices that deliver messages of safety. Beyond breathing exercises, you can try: hugging yourself or another person (gentle thirty-second hugs with someone you trust), slowly rubbing your upper arms or thighs, breathing with your hand on your heart, or splashing cold

water on your face. These techniques have been shown to reduce our response to stress and help with relaxation.[2]

4) A protective vocabulary: Words cannot only help identify a need to slow things down, but also deliver messages of safety. They can be very useful in times when you experience disconnection, escalation, or fear. Sometimes, when we are stressed, there exists an urgency to relieve ourselves of the discomfort. We feel reactive, needing to respond immediately, resolve the issue right away, or run and get as far from the danger as we can. Words like "breathe," "pause," "time out," and "stop" can remind us to take a moment. And in that moment, we can become more expansive in our strategies. Similarly, repeating messages of safety such as "you are safe," "you are not alone," or "you can handle what comes your way" helps your mind relax and reduces muscle tension.

One of our favorite methods for "practicing safety" is to use the Re-STORE method. Every twenty minutes, or every hour, or three times a day, or whatever your preference, use this exercise to build a connection to the language and sensations of safety.

> **Re:** Repeat the following
> **Safe:** I am safe.
> **Time:** There's time.
> **Okay:** Everything is okay.
> **Room:** There is room and freedom.
> **Expansive:** And I can feel the expansiveness right now.

This way, when you are entering a situation that would normally stimulate fear or anxiety, you can repeat this and feel flooded with a sense of safety. The reactive part of your brain, which assesses threats and safety, can't tell time. As such, it will connect with past sensations of safety in the present moment, especially when they arise from familiar, regular, and repeated practices.

Re-STORE method for anticipatory anxiety

Anticipatory anxiety is a fear or worry about something that might happen in the future. Often this is connected to a previous experience or trauma, whether in childhood or adulthood. For example, let's say you had intestinal issues as a child that resulted in frequent visits to the bathroom. Maybe one day you didn't make it in time and had an accident and as a result, even into adulthood, you worry about access to a bathroom. You find yourself feeling overwhelmed or anxious in situations, such as driving in a car or being in an elevator, where you don't have access to a bathroom. Every time you find yourself in these situations, or even think about being in these situations, anticipatory anxiety hits your system and floods it with fear and worry. Instead of succumbing to the anxiety, try to replace it with messages of safety. You can use the Re-STORE method, visualize images, or repeat mantras that help induce calm, peace, and safety. The takeaway here is the bathroom is not the actual issue; the anxiety around it is. In fact, more often than not, the anticipatory fears are much worse than the challenge of actually finding a bathroom.

The more you practice replacing panicked, anxiety-stimulating images with comfortable, safe images that induce calm and peace, the more your body can access the latter in times of need. The key distinction here is that you want to prepare your body (not your brain) by exposing it to anxiety-provoking experiences that you have now enveloped with messages, sensations, and images of safety. Watch your tendency to play out the old unpleasant story or even have fleeting images of negative past experiences. When these arise, you want to retell the story so that it plays out with your desired outcome. For example, "I see myself comfortable and relaxed. My stomach feels settled and I am practicing my Re-STORE to remind myself that I have many options to choose from in the unlikely event that I will need to use the bathroom." The more you can run through this version of the story, not just via words but through feelings and images, the more you will teach your body to feel safe should you find yourself in the situation.

5) Mindfulness: Meditation is one of the more popular avenues for building mindfulness and awareness. If you have an established practice, continue it. For those of you interested in meditation, you can try it on your own or find a guided version that resonates with you. However, meditation is not for everyone. Nor is it the only path to mindfulness. Additional strategies include the Beautiful Flower and Brain vs. Heart.

The Beautiful Flower is particularly enjoyed by children. Imagine that you are a beautiful flower (pick your favorite). A flower retains its beauty in a variety of weather conditions. Like the flower, we, too, remain beautiful as we weather such emotions as joy, sadness, or anger. We are still a beautiful flower even when we make mistakes or show up in less desirable ways. It is in this acceptance that we shift from messages of danger (we are not worthy) to messages of safety (we are enough).

Jordan's beautiful flower

Our daughter drew pictures of every member of our family's beautiful flower. This represents our innate "goodness"; it is always there. We not only have the drawings to refer to, but also the experience of closing our eyes and imagining our beautiful flower. Of course, sometimes we say or do something that stimulates shame. Although our beautiful flower is still there, it temporarily gets covered by fog, making it harder to see. For example, one time our daughter lost her temper and did something that she was really ashamed about. She was super upset and hid her head. We asked her if what she did created fog that made it hard to see her beautiful flower. Because we have practiced this concept already (we regularly take time to check in and see and connect with our beautiful flowers), she was able to track what we were saying. We then asked her if she needed help to support the fog that was coming in and she nodded. One of the things we like to do is sing a song that helps and goes like this:

Jordan is a big, beautiful flower
She's beautiful no matter what she does
Jordan is a big, beautiful flower
Everybody loves Jordan no matter what

Jordan is a big, beautiful flower
She's beautiful no matter what she does
Jordan is a big, beautiful flower
Even if she...

Then we continue by listing anything she can think of that would cause fog:

Even if she... loses her temper and hits her sister because she is really mad
Jordan is a big, beautiful flower

You keep going, trying to flush out anything else she can come up with that would stimulate fog (aka shame) to get it out in the open (where shame can't survive and therefore dissipates):

Even if she... doesn't do something her parents ask
Jordan is a big, beautiful flower

Even if she... calls her sister names because she is angry
Jordan is a big, beautiful flower

The more you list and the sillier they are, the more the shame dissolves and anyone present can add lines, so take turns and have fun:

> *Jordan is a big, beautiful flower*
> *Even if she... picks her nose*
>
> *Jordan is a big, beautiful flower*
> *Even if she... won't eat all of her vegetables*
>
> *Jordan is a big, beautiful flower*
> *Even if she... sneaks candy and cookies without asking*
>
> *Jordan is a big, beautiful flower*
> *Even if she... doesn't do all of her homework*

Eventually you run out of things to add and when that happens you can wrap up the song like this:

> *Jordan is a big, beautiful flower*
> *She's beautiful no matter what she does*
> *Jordan is a big, beautiful flower*
> *Everybody loves Jordan no matter what*

You can end the exercise with a big smile and hug as everyone takes a minute to close their eyes and see their beautiful flower.

Brain vs. heart is a gamified way to notice when we are having inner judgments of blame, shame, guilt, and other unwanted emotions. It works well because it separates our thoughts (brain messages) from our feelings (heart messages). Often, we tend to concern ourselves only with our brain messages. In this state we are unable to tap into our feelings; it is just too vulnerable and risky. As a result, we begin to believe that we are stupid, mean, unlovable, or broken. For example, when we feel shame, we tell ourselves we are worthless. If we don't connect to that feeling, we may begin to believe the message. If we are worthless, who would love us? Does that make us unlovable too? Can you begin to see how traveling down this rabbit hole could make the world around us feel dangerous? The more isolated and alone we become with our thoughts, the more dangerous the world around us seems. By acting out the two "roles," we create a sense of separation and distance that eases us into exploring deeper. This awareness helps us get out of the static state of brain messages (you *are* this or that) to the dynamic state of heart messages (in the moment you *feel* this or that). Releasing the permanence of the former (you are worthless) and stepping into the transience of the latter (you feel shame because you are telling yourself you are worthless) provides a sense of security and safety.

Brain vs. heart with Kylee

The other day our oldest daughter, Kylee (age ten), came home feeling really sad about not being able to understand a new math concept at school. It turned out that her previous school did not teach this concept in a way that enabled her to integrate and apply it. Nevertheless, Kylee was in tears as she tried to figure it out.

As parents, instead of getting angry at her previous teacher or frustrated with Kylee who at this grade level "should" be able to perform these math concepts, we connected to her brain and heart. Her brain was sharing thoughts in the form of judgments and these thoughts were stimulating great pain for her.

By using the brain vs. heart concept, we were able to ask Kylee, what is your brain saying that is hurting your heart's feelings? She shared what we call the "brain message," which was, "The reason I don't know how to do these math problems is because I am stupid!" We then took a moment to feel how much pain and shame were stimulated by this brain message. Working together with her, we translated her brain message to a heart message which sounded like, "I don't know how to do this math problem because I am having trouble comprehending the material and am feeling embarrassed because I want to be more capable as well as have more ease around grasping these concepts."

We took a breath together as she allowed her body to bathe in the compassion and warmth of a heart message. This helped her soften, at which point we were able to empathize with the brain message some more. We wondered together if her brain was trying to help her fit in with the rest of the class, to ensure that she had a sense of belonging as well as skills and abilities that were similar to other kids her age. Kylee agreed with that assessment. Next, we thanked her brain for trying to care for her and protect her and asked that in the future it try to deliver heart messages over judgments. We reminded Kylee to ask for help if her brain was struggling and unable to send messages in a supportive, compassionate, and connecting way. Kylee smiled at the thought of that plan.

What we love about this exercise is that it provides an easy way to not identify with our thoughts and judgments while also not blocking them or judging ourselves for having our judgments. This works well for children and adults... so the next time you catch yourself having a painful brain message, see if you can translate it into a heart message!

The more we feel safe and secure, the easier it is to connect to our authenticity. With the recommendations above, we take the first step, awareness. We now begin to notice what we tell ourselves, the judgments we make, and the feelings that correlate. What often surfaces are needs that have gone unmet for a long time: needs such as worth, security, safety, love, acceptance, predictability, respect, and connection. When we repress these needs, we build up sadness, hurt, fear, anger, resentment, and even rage. Instead of connecting authentically to these feelings and needs, we tell ourselves stories that either blame others (they are mean) or shame us (I don't deserve love, I am stupid, and so forth).

With a connection to our authentic self, we awaken these suppressed and repressed feelings and needs. While initially uncomfortable and possibly even scary, awareness is necessary to begin our healing. The reality is that what we have locked inside affects our health and well-being. Choosing to ignore it doesn't make it disappear. In fact, when we disregard our feelings and needs, we inherently send messages of danger to our brain. As discussed previously, this threat sparks mobilization and a fight-or-flight response that leads to chronic stress and numerous health issues (remember suppression equals inflammation as far as our body is concerned). By practicing messages of safety, we are not only learning to soothe and regulate, but we are also building resilience. We begin to trust that we can care for ourselves, maintaining our health, wellness, and sense of security. There is an understanding that life can be wonderful even with its ups and downs—because we are the ones driving the ship.

In essence, we have the power to determine whether our lives will be wonderful or not by choosing how we respond to our circumstances. We can surrender to our experiences, or we can rewrite our story. And in that revision, we can begin by acknowledging the needs that have been met and those that have not been met. We can celebrate our growth and mourn our losses. We can grieve that our reality is not always what we imagined or hoped it would be. We can come to understand that although we may have preferred certain strategies (our mother's love, to meet needs for self-worth, or our spouse's companionship, to meet needs for warmth), they are not the only option. Our healing allows us to see that we have an abundance of strategies available to meet our needs. For example, we can meet our needs for self-worth externally through friends and work or internally by challenging our negative beliefs, developing and maintaining healthy boundaries, and advocating for ourselves. To meet needs for warmth, we can hang out with a friend, give or get a hug from a loved one, receive empathy, or engage in self-empathy.

There are ample strategies to meet a given need. Yet the only way to find them is to first identify that need. And the only way to uncover the need is to connect to our authentic self and take a personal inventory. We must cultivate the ability to discern so that we can determine what we like and what we don't like, what we want to keep and what we are ready to let go of, what we are feeling and what it tells us about what we are needing. The great news is that we have the answers; we just need to be willing to look within.

CHAPTER 8

Nutrition

Pillar 2

"Those who think they have no time for healthy eating
will sooner or later have to find time for illness."
—EDWARD STANLEY

How do you feel when you hear the word "diet?" It might conjure up a multitude of trendy fads the media bombards us with every couple of years. Or "experts" telling us what we should and shouldn't eat. Suddenly, a food we thought was healthy is off-limits. Or, out of the blue, something is now deemed a "superfood." Who do we believe? How do we know which plan to follow?

This information overload can confuse us, resulting in anxiety, stress, and eventually resignation. It's hard and uncomfortable to diet. And the truth is, it doesn't have to be that complicated.

What if instead of dieting, we start thinking of food as our fuel? If given a choice, wouldn't you choose a fuel that enables you to feel your best, physically and mentally? Wouldn't you want to thrive and feel that Life is Wonderful? Well, guess what, you can and should!

The one thing nearly all popular diet plans agree upon is that whole plant foods are good for you! That is because these are the most nutrient-dense and healthiest foods on the planet.

But there is also a misconception that eating whole plant foods will be tasteless, bland, and boring. No one wants to eat a tasteless and bland meal! We want to enjoy plenty of variety, eat traditional foods at family celebrations, dine out with friends, and indulge during the holidays.

The good news is that you can! You can eat delicious, nutritious food that checks all the boxes without packing on the calories and making yourself sick. And doing so doesn't involve deprivation and restriction. Nor does it mean completely giving up less healthy food choices. Instead, it is about understanding a few simple truths about the foods we eat and then reconfiguring our plates accordingly. Whether you eat to live or live to eat, whole plant foods can meet all your needs.

Simple truth #1: For our ancestors, even though food choices were limited, they were more congruent with health than most of the foods people eat today. They mainly came from whole plants found in nature, which made up most of their caloric intake.

Animal products were scarce and therefore consumed sporadically in small portions. When meat sources were available, the bounty was shared among the village or clan. A little went a long way. And we only ate these higher fat foods occasionally, when the season or location permitted. Imagine climbing a tree in the fall, gathering nuts, and cracking them by hand, rather than having them available 24/7, shelled and ready to eat.

Given the challenges of foraging, food scarcity, changing climates, and difficult terrain, we were a lean and fit species. And we stayed that way, as long as we didn't get eaten by a saber-toothed tiger! The point is that our next meal was not guaranteed. There were no convenience stores and all-day snacking opportunities.

To survive, our bodies need nutrition: foods containing essential nutrients. But many of today's foods contain few nutrients and can be harmful to our bodies. Whole ingredients from nature are manipulated and highly processed into something that hardly resembles our ancestors' fuel and has abnormal effects on our body and brain.

Our body's natural state is to be trim. However, our current environment, particularly the food industry, regularly alters and manipulates our original food sources. Processed foods have replaced whole foods and are abundant everywhere: in corner stores, gas stations, supermarkets, movie theaters, and even health food stores. These convenient options have caused us to crowd out the good stuff with the bad stuff! Most people don't believe this, but the fact is people have to "work" to make their bodies overweight, meaning that the only way to be overweight is to have access to an unnatural food supply. Unfortunately, that "work" is all too easy to do! Thanks to the industrialization of our food supplies, most of the foods we encounter in our grocery stores—outside of the produce aisles—are unnatural, and as a result obesity appears to be our normal state, while being trim and lean appears to be something we have to work hard to achieve.

Simple truth #2: Processed, or packaged, food often removes fiber and water, producing food that no longer resembles its original state (part of the "manipulation" of the food supply). These foods become deficient in essential nutrients after being altered in a factory. They are then fortified and enriched with chemical versions to replace the nutrients lost when processing the whole food. They also contain a laundry list of additives to allow them to live on a shelf for years without spoiling. Just pick up any box of crackers in the supermarket and look at the ingredient list. Unless you live in a science lab, you probably don't keep any of them in your pantry!

On the contrary, whole, unprocessed, and minimally processed plant foods resemble their original state; they spoil quickly and are mainly unpackaged. When packaged, they contain a short, recognizable, and pronounceable list of ingredients. For example, a package of frozen berries contains just berries; crisp bread may contain only whole grain rye flour, yeast, and salt; tomato salsa may contain tomatoes, tomato juice, onions, peppers, herbs, and spices; a package of frozen spinach contains only spinach; and corn tortillas contain just corn, water, and lime. Look for the word "whole" or "stone ground," for example, in bread or flour. It's a good habit to read labels and look for the least number of ingredients, and the most familiar ingredients.

The highly processed, low-grade fuel contains more calories, fat, and salt, and less nutrients and fiber. We use the term calorie-dense to describe these foods that pack a high caloric load per unit of weight. Like processed foods, meat and dairy are also calorie-dense options. In addition, processed foods and animal products also contain more environmental contaminants. In the case of processed foods, this comes from preservatives, flavorings, and colorings; in animal products, it's the result of a process (biomagnification) that we will explain momentarily.

You may be asking yourself at this point, if the environment is so polluted with chemicals, don't the plants take them up as well? The answer is yes; unfortunately, the plants will absorb some of those chemicals. (Or they may not, especially if the plants are grown organically.) BUT—and this is a big but—they absorb them in much smaller amounts than do, for example, fish. The reason for this is twofold: first, plants are low in fat, and these chemicals are lipophilic (meaning they like to hide in fat). Second, plants are low on the food chain, while animals are high on the food chain. Through the process known as biomagnification, the higher up on the food chain something is, the more toxicity it carries. A plant may absorb, let's say, five units (parts per million) of these chemicals. Fish eat many plants, and for *each* one they eat, they get five units; this is the process of magnification. The fish then store these contaminants in their body. When larger fish eat smaller fish, these toxins get concentrated. By the time we eat the fish, they have accumulated a large amount of these toxic contaminants.

We, like the animals, also store these toxins in our bodies. The only way to get rid of them is by eliminating them from our diet and allowing them to break down over time. For example, dioxin, one of the most carcinogenic environmental toxins that exists, has a half-life of seven years. In other words, if we had 100 fgs (femtograms) of dioxin in our bodies today and did not consume any more of it, then in seven years we would bring that level down to 50 fgs and in another seven years we would be down to 25 fgs, and so on. It is worth noting that the Environmental Protection Agency says that 93% of our dioxin exposure comes from consuming animal products, in particular fish and dairy.[1]

Most people desire to live a long and healthy life. If that is important to you, then studies show that "Increasing intakes of healthy plant foods and decreasing intakes of less healthy plant or animal foods can lower the future risk of mortality."[2] This study found that processed plant foods increased the risk of death, meaning that not all foods derived from plants are created equal. If you eat a whole plant food that is unprocessed or minimally processed, then you will increase your longevity, but if you consume processed "junk" plant foods, then you will decrease your longevity. And for those who are afraid of carbohydrates, it is important to note that decreasing them may be concerning too. That is because limiting carbohydrates includes reducing the health-promoting whole plant food varieties (fruits, vegetables, whole grains, legumes, and some nuts and seeds) and not just the junk carbs. In fact, one study looked at nearly 25,000 people following low carb diets over 6.4 years and found that "participants with the LOWEST carbohydrates intake had the HIGHEST risk of overall, cardiovascular disease, cerebrovascular, and cancer mortality."[3] This means that blanket condemnation of carbohydrates can harm your health whereas in-

Examples of Health Promoting vs. Non-Health Promoting Foods
Health Promoting
Fruits: melons, bananas, apples, pears, berries
Vegetables: broccoli, cauliflower, kale, spinach, peppers, artichoke, cucumbers
Whole grains: millet, oats, quinoa, rice
Starchy vegetables: sweet and regular potatoes, corn, squash
Legumes: lentils, beans, split peas
Nuts and seeds: sunflower seeds, almonds, walnuts
Non-Health Promoting
Ultra-processed and refined food-like substances: cakes, cookies, candies, chips (potato, tortilla, etc.), pretzels, chocolate bars, many fast-food options (like hot dogs, burgers, donuts), soft drinks, isolated macronutrients (whey protein, soy protein, pea protein, fiber), oil, and sugar
Animal products: All meats, fish, eggs, cheeses, and dairy

clusion of healthy whole carbohydrates can significantly benefit your health and reduce your risk of early mortality. So be careful not to throw the baby out with the bathwater when you think of carbohydrates in the future.

Whole plant foods are high in vitamins, minerals, antioxidants, and other phytochemicals that contribute to our health, and they are low in environmental contaminants. They contribute to weight loss and prevent obesity because most are low in calories (calorie-dilute) and high in nutrients. Additionally, whole plant foods reduce and can often reverse the risk of major diseases, including today's most common: heart disease, diabetes, autoimmune disorders, inflammation, and cancer.

Understanding the two simple truths discussed above helps us see that our current environment is not prioritizing health promoting foods. Processed, calorie-dense foods are abundant, advertised, and easily accessed. It is no surprise that we gravitate towards them.

Simple truth #3: Calorie density simply means the number of calories in a given weight of food. Whole, unprocessed plant foods are the lowest in calorie density and therefore calorie dilute. You can eat more, because they properly regulate hunger signals by giving us the bulk (nutrients, water, and fiber) we need. Our stomachs stretch appropriately and give our brains the message that we have consumed the necessary number of calories. Thus, the brain and gut are in sync. Eating in the optimal caloric density range fills us with just the right number of calories and prevents overconsumption or weight gain. For example, a pound of broccoli is about 100-200 calories whereas a pound of crackers is about 2,250 calories. You probably wouldn't sit down and eat pounds of broccoli, because its bulk (fiber, water, nutrients) would fill you up before you could eat that much.

On the contrary, processed foods have few nutrients and have removed much of the water and fiber, thus becoming calorie-dense. A little bit of processed food packs a high caloric load. The more calorie-dense a portion of food, the easier it is to overeat by consuming more calories than your body actually needs. Eating just a small portion will leave you hungry, so to feel satisfied you will continue eating more calories than you need. Lacking fiber, nutrients, and water, calorie-dense foods such as crackers and cheese do not have the bulk to stretch our stomachs appropriately; therefore, our brain doesn't get the message that we've had enough. This lack of synchronization confuses the brain, and we "trust our gut," which, in this case, unfortunately, leads us to overconsumption of calories.

If you enjoy eating, but want to maintain a healthy weight, think of it this way: when you eat calorie-dense foods, you get to eat only a fraction of the amount of food that you can eat when you eat whole plant foods, if you want to eat the same number of calories.

Caloric Density	
Raw Veggies	100-200 calories/pound
Fruits	200-400 calories/pound
Starchy veggies	300-400 calories/pound
Whole grains	400-500 calories/pound
Legumes	500-600 calories/pound
Avocado	750 calories/pound
Animal Products	700-1200 calories/pound
Pure Sugar	1800 calories/pound
Chocolate	2200 calories/pound
Cookies	2250 calories/pound
Nuts/Seeds	2600 calories/pound
Oils	4000 calories/pound

The goal (for optimum health and weight) for the average person is to minimize (or eliminate, especially if the goal is weight loss) the foods that are over 600 calories per pound. Notice how most whole foods (exceptions are nuts, seeds, and avocados) naturally average in that calorie density "sweet spot," while processed foods and animal products do not. It is important to note, especially for those trying to lose weight, that although nuts, seeds, and avocados are healthy choices, they should be consumed in smaller portions (particularly for those who are trying to lose weight) because they are more calorie-dense. On the other hand, athletes might take advantage of calorie-dense foods to try to keep up with their exceptionally high metabolism.

When we hiked up Mt. Whitney and could only carry so much food in our backpack, we included more calorie-dense foods such as dried fruits and nuts, in order to be able to maximize calories in a relatively small space (our backpacks). So, you can see how calorie density should not be thought of as "good" or "bad"; it varies with the situation. Most people in today's society, however, consume too many calories already and consequently struggle with extra weight. For this group, especially if weight loss is desired, aiming to lower their average calorie density would be beneficial.

Simple truth #4: We are getting sicker and much of that is attributable to the foods we eat on a daily basis.

- 50% of American adults have a preventable diet and lifestyle-related chronic disease: heart disease, high blood pressure, diabetes, autoimmune conditions, and some cancers.[4]
- Every thirty-seven seconds in America, someone dies of heart disease.[5]
- One in three Americans born in 2000 will develop diabetes in their lifetime.[6]
- "Approximately 40% of children had intermediate or poor total cholesterol levels," in a study looking at nearly 9000 children.[7]
- Over two-thirds of adults and one-third of children are overweight or obese. This increases risk for diabetes, heart disease, high blood pressure, arthritis-related conditions, and cancer.[8]

Alona's story—A plant-based diet reversed my aunt's heart disease

My aunt had a history of yo-yo dieting. She would lose thirty, forty, even fifty pounds, only to gain them back again and then some. I had shared with her the many benefits of plant-based eating, everything from health (disease prevention and reversal) to the ability to eat without restriction and deprivation. Despite knowing the information, she wasn't interested. Not even when she got diagnosed with high blood pressure and elevated cholesterol. Her preference was to take medication that would "resolve" her health issues. That was the case until she had a heart attack when she turned sixty. It turned out she had one artery that was 90% blocked and another that was 70% blocked. Her doctor stented the first one and decided to wait three weeks to stent the second.

It was then that I got the call: "I will do whatever you tell me, just please help." I put my aunt on a 100% whole foods plant-based diet. For the three weeks leading up to her procedure, we put together a meal plan that incorporated a variety of recipes and even included desserts. She followed the plan faithfully and after weeks went back to see her doctor. As they prepped for the procedure, the doctor was shocked to find that her 70% blockage had decreased to 45%! My aunt no longer needed a second stent. Learning about the changes she had made, her doctor replied, "Keep doing whatever you are doing, it is obviously working."

Simple truth #5: Willpower doesn't work. It is a losing battle to continue to eat the same foods that have made you overweight and sick, and simply try to restrict their quantity. Restriction confuses our brain into thinking we are starving. Our instinct to survive overpowers our will to restrict and eventually leads to overeating and even bingeing. Therefore, reliance on willpower and yo-yoing (from eating enough to not eating enough) are short-term strategies that almost always fail. The best way to avoid this trap is by reconfiguring our plate to include more fruits, vegetables, whole grains, and legumes so that most of our diet is composed of foods with a calorie density of 600 or less. In this way, we get calorie-dilute and nutrient-rich food that contains enough bulk to appropriately shut off hunger signals, keeping us satisfied while preventing overeating and weight gain.

A large portion of the bulk provided in whole plant-based foods comes from fiber. When we speak of fiber, we are not talking about your grandparents' bran muffins and fiber supplements, but the fiber that's intrinsic to whole, unprocessed plant foods. Fiber promotes bowel regularity, feeds our healthy gut flora, stabilizes our blood sugar, and helps eliminate unwanted hormones and toxins. Thanks to that fiber, whole food fuel sources naturally keep us trim like our ancestors because they fill us up and regulate hunger signals. The nutrients, water, and fiber (bulk) give our brains and stomachs the message that we have consumed just enough food to be satiated, and we can stop eating.

Sadly, this is not so for the majority of the foods that many of us eat. Did you ever wonder why it's so hard to stop eating that piece of cake, chocolate chip cookies, or ice cream? It just feels so good. Well, it's due to the chemical called dopamine your brain releases when you experience something pleasurable. Eating, intimacy, and certain drugs like heroin and morphine give you a dopamine hit. Processed food manufacturers engineer their products to do exactly the same thing, making their potato chips, pretzels, and cookies as addictive as opiates.

Eating higher-calorie foods gives us a greater dopamine hit. This signal was an evolutionary advantage when food was scarce and in short supply, and, in order to conserve energy, we needed to spend less time searching for it. We were drawn to the calorie-dense foods that helped decrease the number of times we would have to risk our lives foraging for food. Today, our bodies still "reward" us (via dopamine) for choosing the most calorie-dense foods even though obtaining those foods no longer poses a risk to our survival. In fact, today's calorie-dense imposter foods trick us and keep us trapped in an unhealthy cycle that has replaced the risk to our survival.

Eating highly processed, calorie-dense foods and receiving higher dopamine hits raises our baseline. Over time, as with drugs, we build up a tolerance and need even higher-calorie foods to be satisfied. So eventually, the higher dopamine hits become a new baseline. We need to eat more to get that next dopamine hit. And the cycle continues. But we can break the cycle!

You know how when you walk into a dark movie theater, you can't see? Then after a minute or two, your eyes adjust, and you can suddenly see well enough to find your seat. That's called neural adaptation. Or in the case of someone changing from coffee to decaf or refined to whole grain: at first, this may feel uncomfortable. But the brain and body adapt quickly to a new normal. If only we trusted that, making changes would be so much easier.

For many people who adopt plant-based eating, the most difficult food to give up is cheese. For some, it is the last to go; for others, it is a dealbreaker. Why is it so difficult to cut out cheese? All mother's milk contains a protein called casein that contains casomorphin, a compound that works much like an opiate in our system by triggering the pleasure chemical dopamine. It's one of nature's miracles: for a baby animal to thrive, it must be "addicted" to its mother's milk. But once an animal is old enough, it weans from its mother's milk to eat solid food. Humans' consumption of dairy products prolongs that "addiction" to the casomorphin we consume from cow, goat, and sheep's milk, and therefore we are never truly weaned.

Unfortunately, cheese is one of the most highly processed foods out there. It is pasteurized, fermented by bacteria, coagulated with enzymes, separated into solids, salted, and aged. Like other dairy products, it is also high in saturated fats and is very calorie-dense. It also stimulates the secretion of IGF-1 (insulin-like growth factor), a chemical compound that is great for stimulating quick growth for baby cows into large adult cows but not at all helpful when it stimulates the same rapid growth for cancer or promotes premature aging.[9] Dairy contributes to weight gain, heart disease, diabetes, and autoimmune disorders.[10] As with meat, which has a similar profile, it is best to consume it in very small portions or infrequently, if at all.

But if I limit dairy and meat, you may ask, where will I get my protein? We don't know about you, but we have never met anyone who suffers from kwashiorkor. Never heard of it? It's the name for protein deficiency. You've never heard of it because kwashiorkor is extremely rare in developed countries (people with protein deficiency in developing nations are not just deficient in protein, but completely malnourished).

Even so, misinformation has led us to obsess over getting enough protein. We are scared into believing we need to eat meat to get enough; therefore, we over-consume it, which is one of the reasons why heart disease remains the number one killer in America. All animals, including humans, make cholesterol. When we eat animals, we essentially eat their cholesterol, adding to our own. As a result, we accumulate more than our bodies can process. And since animal protein contains no fiber, the body struggles to assimilate the fat and cholesterol: a recipe for heart disease and strokes.

Whole plant foods provide all the macro and micronutrients we need to thrive and contain all the essential amino acids (those we need to consume because we cannot make them) that make up protein. Ideally, whole plant foods should (and could!) make up the foundation of your diet. Fruits, vegetables, starchy vegetables, whole grains, and legumes—along with some nuts and seeds—are the most nutrient-rich food groups. They're low in fat, yet offer all the essential fatty acids; they have low caloric density, yet are satiating so that you will feel satisfied and remain trim without caloric restriction; and they do not contain any cholesterol (we can make all of the cholesterol we need without consuming it in our diet).

Supplements

Whenever possible, eat the nutrients you need from the source rather than supplementing with a pill. Nutrients delivered from whole foods are readily available and delivered in bal-

anced quantities. Supplements, on the other hand, are artificial, manipulated, and often isolated so that the nutrients they contain function individually in our bodies rather than in conjunction with other nutrients. Relying on supplements to supply your nutrient needs would be like trying to drive your car with just a steering wheel, tire, and/or windshield. Eating a diet rich in whole plant foods supplies a balanced variety of nutrients that we need in their appropriate proportions. This allows our body to accurately metabolize them for optimal functioning. Supplements, on the other hand, arrive separately and in artificial forms and amounts with dosages often higher than we need. Science has shown that the premise that "more is better" is not true. What results with supplemented nutrients is an imbalance in integration and distribution, resulting in a different, and sometimes even harmful, impact compared to its natural counterpart (whole foods). For example, excess iron supplementation can damage the stomach, the digestive tract, and the liver.[11] Overconsumption of calcium is associated with an increased risk of heart attack, stroke, kidney damage, and death.[12] Excess magnesium can lead to muscle weakness and heart damage.[13] And the list goes on. Other than B12 supplementation (which is needed by many people, including vegans and vegetarians), it is increasingly unlikely that there are any long-term benefits of supplementation that outweigh the known and unknown risks. As such, we should take care not to supplement simply as a means of negating unhealthy eating habits or as an "insurance policy." If you are truly deficient or unable to obtain, absorb, or metabolize nutrients from food, then supplementation could be indicated. However, as doctors, we would still want to work with you to determine what is causing these underlying issues and ideally restore your natural ability to obtain nutrients from food. Ultimately, it's best to discuss the risks and benefits of supplementation with a physician you trust.

The question at mealtime shouldn't be, *"Will I get enough protein?"* but rather, *"Am I getting enough fiber?!"*

We often hear, *but beans give me gas!* Sometimes switching to whole plant foods initially can cause bloating and flatulence. Our digestive systems need to adapt to these unprocessed foods that haven't been broken down for us by machines. Mastication, or chewing our food, is how we break it down, and during that process, the food mixes with enzymes in our mouths, and when it gets to our digestive system fills us up and feeds the microbiome, or healthy flora. As the microbiome improves, the gas subsides. Yet we eat standing up, while working, on the run, or in the car, rush through our meals, and aren't paying attention to how we are eating, when what we need is to slow down, relax at mealtime, and chew and enjoy our food. The more you can be present and focus on the food, the more you will distinguish its flavors, fill up faster, and eat less.

There is a story about a Zen meditation teacher who gave each of his students one potato chip and instructed them to chew very slowly until the potato chip was liquid in their mouths before they swallowed it. The students were very excited but complained they didn't think they could "eat just one." However, they complied and spent several minutes sitting on their cushions with their eyes closed, crunching, and savoring one chip. Many of the students were surprised at their experience and reported the overwhelming and off-putting flavor of salt and grease and discovered eating the chip this way made it distasteful. The students concluded if they were watching TV and mindlessly snacking, they could see how easy it would be to eat the whole bag.

People eat for many reasons, but here are five leading ones:

1. Hunger
2. Boredom
3. Stress
4. Fatigue
5. It's available

To help you with why you eat, try this test:

On a scale of 1-10, rate how hungry you are, and then on another scale from 1-10, rate how much you want the food. The difference between those two numbers is all the other reasons you are eating that don't have to do with a genuine need for food.

What if you changed your way of dealing with the five incentives to eat in the following way:

You are hungry: eat until comfortably full.
You are bored: play a game, call a friend, or engage in a fun activity.
You feel stressed: take a walk, do deep breathing, or stretch.
You feel fatigued: take a nap, and if you can't, try 5-10 jumping jacks.
Food is available: keep only whole plant foods in your kitchen and environment!

To make nutrition changes, it is essential to identify your needs. In this way, you can ensure that your strategies meet all your needs and not some at the expense of others.

But how do you do this?

Build habits that eliminate decision fatigue. Instead of getting overwhelmed and trying to plan for three meals a day, seven days a week, keep it simple. Find two or three healthy, whole plant food dishes you could enjoy at each mealtime. Then rotate them throughout the week for breakfast, lunch, dinner, and snacks. Ideally, aim for 80-100% whole plant-based foods and no more than 20% discretionary.

Most importantly, don't focus on what you can't eat. Instead, focus on what you can by adding less calorie-dense foods! To each meal, add as many low-calorie, low-fat, and high-nutrient foods as you can. This process of adding healthy, nutrient-rich foods will prevent you from feeling deprived and keep you focused on all that you can have.

As you add to your meals and incorporate these whole plant foods, your taste buds begin to adapt, enabling you to focus on limiting or removing (crowding out) the amount of high-calorie, high-fat, and low-nutrient foods you consume.

When you are cooking at home, get creative! Use your favorite herbs and spices liberally to keep your taste buds happy. And when eating out and shopping, seek plant-based versions of your favorite dishes: dairy-free spinach lasagna, loaded veggie pizza hold-the-cheese, tofu stir fry, bean burritos, veggie burgers, and pasta marinara. It's easier than ever to find delicious and healthier versions of them all! The plant-based movement is becoming more and more popular in restaurants and markets worldwide.

Forget willpower, moderation, deprivation, fasting, and the confusing quick-fix methods for changing your dietary habits—none of these approaches is sustainable. Instead, aim to begin with small changes in your daily meals. It's better to be excited about changing five meals in your week than feel overwhelmed trying to change everything. Once those small changes become routine, keep evolving your plate until you have reached your ratio of at least 80/20.

It's much easier than you think! Here are some tips:

1. Create a meal plan for diversity and satiation: think about those two or three meals you can incorporate into your week. For example: oatmeal, potato hash, or pancakes for breakfast; bean and veggie burrito or baked potato stuffed with veggie chili along with a salad for lunch; and whole grain pasta with marinara or a black bean burger and salad for dinner. Healthy snacks such as apples or bananas with a little nut butter, rice cakes with guacamole, potato wedges with ketchup, or carrots and hummus are great to have on hand. And to stave off sweet tooth cravings, include desserts such as fruit salad, baked apple, or nuts and date truffles.
   Remember, keep it simple!
2. Allow for eating out: many restaurants have various options of dishes that are easily adaptable to meet your dietary needs. It helps to look at the menu ahead of time. These days, it is very likely they will offer a vegan (though not always a whole food)

option. Many restaurants will accommodate omitting or limiting oil in a dish (remember, oil is highest on the calorie density chart). There are almost always salads and sides to bulk up your plate or create a delicious meal.

3. Acknowledge your "deal-breakers" upfront and leave them alone —everything else is fair game! For instance, "I could never go plant based because I would never give up half-and-half in my coffee." If that's your deal breaker, then don't allow it to prevent you from changing all of your other dietary habits. Keep it in the mix. Have your half-and-half in your coffee and focus on other areas you know could use improvement, such as adding more whole plant foods to your meals. Once you do so, it may eventually feel natural to play with modifying the deal-breaker (e.g., finding a plant-based creamer).

4. Eat low on the calorie density scale, especially when building your new taste buds. This means starting with mostly low-calorie-dense foods and then adding small amounts of more-calorie-dense items. Remember to focus on eating foods with a calorie density of 600 or less.

5. Another great trick is to begin your meals by first eating whole foods, such as an apple or your favorite fruit or vegetable or a potato! Choose the low-calorie density foods first and then eat the rest of the meal. (This is important because once you eat the higher density foods that release more dopamine, it will be harder to go back to lower calorie density foods.) Studies show that people who eat whole, lower calorie foods first consume fewer calories at mealtime.

As the famous saying goes, the journey of a thousand miles begins with a single step. Perhaps now your journey to a vibrant self will begin with a single serving. Focus on whole plant foods and evolve your plate, one bite at a time.

		FIBER	WATER	FAT
Lower calorie density, high nutrient foods (100-600 range)	Fruits	HIGH	HIGH	LOW
	Vegetables	HIGH	HIGH	LOW
	Legumes	HIGH	HIGH	LOW
	Complex grains & starches	HIGH	HIGH	LOW
Higher calorie density, low nutrient foods (700-4000 range)	Animal foods	NONE	LESS	HIGH
	Oils	NONE	NONE	HIGH
	Ultra-processed foods	LITTLE to NONE	LITTLE to NONE	HIGH

What about my family?

Some people might be thinking: "It's hard enough to change my own diet but how do I get my family to eat this way, too?" Good question! In our home, we attempt to care about everyone's needs using compassionate communication (more on this in Chapters 12 and 13), which means we try to respect choices around food. Recently our daughter Kylee, 10, came home from school and asked why she has to be vegan. Instead of answering her question, we first empathized with what we believed were the underlying needs stimulating that question.

"Kylee, are you feeling disappointed because you really want to fit in with your friends at school and have the meals you eat look similar to the meals your friends eat?"

Kylee answered with a resounding "YES! I always bring stuff that looks so different from what my friends are eating."

We continued with "And maybe you are needing more ease and harmony at school and feel hurt and sad if someone makes fun of you for being vegan?"

She responded, looking down and nodding her head.

We spent a little more time connecting around the pain stimulated in her at school, and as she processed, we asked if she just wanted to be heard or if she had room to hear our reaction. She said she appreciated being heard and then did want to hear our reaction. We explained that we, too, value her feeling ease and flow in school and experiencing a sense of belonging and acceptance. We also value her autonomy and choice around what feels right to her and what is in integrity with her values. Finally, we said that we trust she cares about her health and well-being, as well as the well-being of other animals and life on this planet, including the environment. She nodded in agreement, at which point we agreed to figure out how what she eats impacts all of those needs.

We said, "Kylee, first we don't want you to feel forced into any decision. In other words, we want you to choose exactly what you want to eat. Second, we want you to be prepared to stand up for yourself, whatever you choose to eat, to ensure you meet your needs for self-respect and dignity. Hearing that, do you want to make changes to your diet now or wait until you explore all of the information and then make changes? We can support you either way."

This last point is important because what she chooses to eat in the next few days, weeks, or months really won't have much impact in the grand scheme of her life. Making that clear to her immediately gave her a choice, which felt wonderful to her.

Ultimately, Kylee decided to not make changes to her vegan diet, while she was still gathering information, but rather to choose different meals for lunch at school. To help meet her needs for belonging, we created a new menu including peanut butter and jelly sandwiches, pasta, and rice and beans with tortilla chips. We also engaged in some role playing to help empower her when schoolmates commented on her lunch. Kylee listed all *of the things other kids said that stimulated hurt and discomfort, and we role-played things she could say in response.*

Ultimately, Kylee was able to choose what to eat and discovered ways to meet her needs for self-respect and dignity. Suddenly, dissatisfaction and urgency for change were replaced with choice, comfort, and empowerment. We closed the loop to provide the additional information she was curious about, by watching several documentaries on various topics, including animal agriculture, ethics, health, and the environment. Kylee landed on wanting to remain vegan, but now she was vegan because she wanted to be, not because her parents were vegan or forced her to be vegan. She was armed with information to share with her friends if they were truly curious about her choices and she was empowered with ways to address those who made comments, so she didn't internalize insults but instead stood up for herself with strength and compassion. When we take this approach to connect to people's underlying needs instead of being attached to a particular strategy (like obedience or conformity), everyone thrives and Life is Wonderful!

Last points to consider

For those of you struggling with your diet, or who have perhaps tried and failed to make dietary changes or to achieve sustained weight-loss, here are three things to consider that might provide some light and self-compassion for your current situation and previous challenges:

1) Learned helplessness

Learned helplessness is a term that was coined by Martin Seligman. He found that dogs who were exposed to painful electrical shocks while locked in their cage, unable to free themselves, had become victims of learned helplessness. In other words, these dogs learned that they couldn't free themselves, so even when the door was open to the half of the cage where there was no electric shock being given, they continued to lay there getting shocked. However, dogs that were not exposed to the shocks while locked in the cage immediately ran to the safe side of the cage when the door was opened. The only way to get the original dogs to overcome their learned helplessness was to drag them out so that they could physically experience the path to freedom.

This experiment was exceedingly cruel and we do not condone this form of animal experimentation. Nonetheless, since it is now part of scientific literature and hopefully will not be repeated, there are lessons we can learn from it.

Many of us have been locked in a nutritional cage, enduring all sorts of pain, not knowing how to free ourselves. For example, there is the pain of fear of the food tasting bad, the discomfort of restriction and portion control, the fear of protein deficiency, or the social isolation of eating differently. Now with the information in this book, we are opening the door to the cage you have endured for so long. But just like the dogs in the experiment, you may be a victim of learned helplessness so that even intellectual understanding of this path to freedom will not be enough. People who have experienced this type of pain in their lives, unable to free themselves from that pain, rarely take the path to freedom if there is only intellectual understanding. In fact, we often choose to stay in the fear and pain we know rather than "risk" the unknown or the pain of failure from trying and not succeeding. As a result, to achieve change you must be "dragged" out of your cage so that you can physically experience the path to freedom and know what it feels like to be free from a lifetime of struggles with diet and lifestyle changes. Much of the work we do at WeHeal, with clients individually and in groups, is to support and encourage this "dragging" towards freedom.

2) Life otherwise stinks

If your life stinks, then addiction (to food, alcohol, drugs, and other tragic habits) might be the only sources of "pleasure" you may have. We say "pleasure" because of the huge cost that it comes with, as addiction cannot bring true joy. In the world of nutrition, the Standard American Diet (S.A.D.) with its abundance of highly processed, high-fat, high-salt, and high-sugar foods, often serves as a "drug" providing some pleasure in a life that offers little to no other sources of joy. When people have nothing to look forward to in their lives other than some dopamine hits from the foods they choose, then it makes sense not to want to give that up. Sometimes you have to address other life factors before changing your diet.

That is where the EoW pillars come in. At WeHeal, we use these pillars to identify where you need the most attention and support, begin there, and then branch out to the other areas of your life that you wish to change. Maybe you need to address sleep deprivation, your disconnection with your partner or boss, or years of suppressing and repressing your true self, before attempting to change your diet. The empowerment here is in awareness. If you insist on making changes to your diet without working on other more pressing issues, you may continue to fail and ultimately feel hopeless. On the other hand, understanding that these issues are present and need to be addressed before, or in conjunction with, dietary changes, will help you feel encouraged and optimistic.

3) Lack of clarity

You may not know what Life Is Wonderful even looks like. Like the dogs who became victims of learned helplessness, you need to be physically exposed to what a joyful life could be to know what it feels like in your body and to truly believe it is possible. You need to shift how you view your world and discern what you do want out of every moment, hour, day, week, month, and year.

The clearer you can get, the more likely you will be to make this shift. Your brain defaults to where you put your energy most. If you are always focused on what isn't working, what you don't like, and how dangerous and scary the world is, then that is how your brain will scan the world, looking for proof to support those beliefs. Instead, we can start focusing on what is working (the actions that have met our needs in the past, so we can reinforce them), what we do like, how the world may be a safer place than we think, and the knowledge that you have skills to navigate it even when there are moments of concern and worry. In other words, shift your intention and the way you show up in every moment so that your brain defaults to looking for proof that your Life Is Wonderful!

You may need to ask yourself if you need help to "drag" you out of your current diet and lifestyle, in order to arrive at a felt, physical experience of that path to freedom to truly know that it is possible.

CHAPTER 9

Activity

Pillar 3

"Take care of your body. It's the
only place you have to live."

—JIM ROHN

WITH NATIONAL FITNESS CHAINS, home gym equipment, spin studios, yoga studios, and outdoor workout clubs, exercise has never been more accessible. But between our full-time jobs, school, kids, and other daily demands, it's hard to imagine making the time for yet one more thing.

We dread the time it takes to plan the round-trip drive to the fitness center. Then we spend an hour conjuring up energy we don't have, all to do something we may not enjoy. And it costs money. But we hear it constantly: exercise is essential for our health and well-being. Some of us punish our bodies into submission, while others don't make it a priority at all. It's no wonder exercise can be so daunting.

But why is exercise so important? Why is fitness a billion-dollar industry? Because study after study shows that physical activity decreases disease risk, including high blood pressure, diabetes, cancer, and osteoporosis. Yet our environment no longer supports or provides many opportunities for movement.

Historically, people did not formally exercise. Instead, movement was incorporated into their everyday lives. Even as recently as two hundred years ago, 90% of the world lived in agricultural communities.

People sat for only three to five hours daily and mostly to take breaks from work. Modern Americans sit for 13 to 15 hours per day![1]

Exercise may be a strategy, but movement is a universal need.

Nowadays, if our job or lifestyle doesn't require or naturally include regular physical activity, we must create ways to move our bodies. Structured exercise is the modern person's equivalent of nutritional supplements. Just as supplements should not be the bulk of your diet, structured exercise should not be the bulk of your movement profile. Unless, of course, you are a professional athlete.

Many of us spend an hour at the gym or commit to structured exercise before or after work. The rest of the time, we sit at our desks or in front of our televisions and computers. Even those of us with excellent exercise habits spend most of our non-exercise time not moving. When we've checked the exercise box, we perceive ourselves as active, but the almost-all-day stillness is the problem. Movement is crucial for humans.

Sadly, modern life has removed the need to move frequently every day. We get up, get into our cars, find the closest parking spot to our destination, and take the elevator up to our office.

At home, we've got robot vacuum cleaners and remote-controlled devices, automated lights, garage door openers, motion sensor gates, and the like. It's no longer even necessary to go to the store. We can order anything we need online from the comfort of our recliner, including groceries delivered to our door. Thus, for many of us, daily life requires minimal movement.

A sedentary lifestyle has a huge cost. Excessive sitting is associated with a number of diseases and conditions, including back pain, obesity, cardiovascular disease, hypertension, cancer, and depression. In contrast, almost every disease lists "exercise" as a preventive or therapeutic treatment.

While "being sedentary" is often assumed to mean the opposite of "being an exerciser," sedentarism is determined by your most frequent behavior, not by brief periods of your most intense. Examples of sedentary activities, as listed in the Journal of the Academy of Nutrition and Dietetics, include sitting, lying down, watching TV, using the computer, reading, and sleeping.

People who are regularly physically active have a lower risk of all-cause mortality compared to physically inactive people. Regular exercise increases your metabolic rate, which will burn more calories and support weight loss efforts. The degree and type of external movement directly impact cardiovascular function, muscle development, hormones, and every other body system. Activity is required to pump lymph throughout the body (helping to excrete toxins, viruses, bacteria, and cells that can cause cancer) and aid blood return from the extremities (important for maintaining good circulation). The movement of blood, nutrients, oxygen, and cellular energy depends on being physically active. Also, exercise helps build bone density when you're younger, helping to prevent osteoporosis later in life.

We have a lot of excuses for not moving and exercising, so it may be helpful to identify top obstacles. One obstacle is inability to afford a gym membership. Fortunately, exercise can take many forms that do not require a gym membership. Lack of time is another obstacle. The good news: you don't have to exercise for long bursts of time.

Now let's look at the possible opportunities to bring movement into our lives. Since physical activity of any kind will benefit your health, think of creative ways to make it part of your daily routine. We can create movement in our day, no matter what we are wearing or where we happen to be. For instance, choose the farthest parking space from the office or grocery store, take walking breaks instead of coffee breaks, walk stairs instead of using the elevator, and get your heart rate up with housework by pumping up some rockin' music and picking up the pace. There are many free videos online for chair yoga at your desk, five-minute office workouts, or how to use our environment as our gym so that we can get our exercise in without fancy equipment. Running/jogging/walking outdoors, jumping rope, dancing, yoga in the park, hiking, biking, kayaking, rowing, roller skating, and swimming are all wonderful ways people enjoy moving their bodies. It won't be so daunting if we allow ourselves to build the activity we enjoy into our day. The key is to find the way you love to move and do more of that... every day!

Many of us fall into the all-or-nothing trap. If we don't commit to an hour of exercise, then we forego it all together. We forget that what's more important is fitting in short bursts several times a day. Start slow and build up. You don't need to begin by running a marathon. Instead, take a five-to-ten minute walk around the neighborhood, do ten jumping jacks, or other light exercise. Stick with your five or ten minutes a day, and when it becomes routine, tack on another five or ten.

Some ideas for those at work: consider standing desks, balance boards, yoga balls as chairs, and treadmills. These are great ways to stay active while working at your computer or on a long conference call. They don't require getting sweaty and breathless but do provide you with low impact, steady movement, and muscle engagement instead of being sedentary for hours on end.

There is accumulating data showing that High Intensity Interval Training (HIIT) is a valuable source of cardiovascular health and may also have additional benefits at the mitochondrial level (the energy factories within your cells), including restorative and regenerative impacts on the body and unique impacts on chronic disease. Research "demonstrates that high-intensity interval training (HIT) can serve as an effective alternate to traditional endurance-based training, inducing similar or even superior physiological adaptations in healthy individuals and diseased populations…"[2]

For those who are able to do so safely, slowly working up to the addition of HIIT may be of additional value to your activity regimen. This is all still being studied, but short duration HIIT has comparable benefits to moderate-intensity continuous training despite significantly lower time commitments. Given that "lack of time" remains the most commonly cited barrier to regular exercise, this may be a wonderful option for some. And for those who enjoy taking advantage of all the potential health benefits, there seems to be little risk (if worked up to safely) of adding HIIT to your cardiovascular exercise regimen. This might include, for example, working up to five thirty-second bursts of high intensity running as fast and hard as you can (interwoven with thirty seconds of walking) during the midpoint of a run. The key is starting slowly and working your way up with HIIT, as the only thing worse than not exercising is injuring yourself while exercising!

Although high intensity interval training has its value, movement and exercise do not have to be intense to offer benefits. Avoiding high intensity exercise does reduce (for some more than others) the risk of injury. Additionally, lower intensity activity keeps our bodies in an aerobic energy-burning state (oxygen-requiring). We increase our heart and breathing rates to provide more oxygen to our muscles. Because this exercise is less intense, you can sustain it longer, thereby continuing to burn fat and contributing to weight loss. High intensity exercise is too vigorous to depend on the burning of oxygen alone. Instead, the preferred fuel is derived from breaking down energy (glycogen) already stored in your muscles; in addition, fat is also burned.

Movement and exercise use various muscle groups. A person's strength is based on the load that a muscle can hold or endure. Strength is developed and maintained by engaging muscles in activities that work and train them to hold, carry, or lift increasing amounts of weight. Using all the muscle groups is essential to help strengthen all the little supporting muscles we need for good posture. We need to move our bodies regularly to maintain the ability to move through life with ease.

To a large degree, your body requires that you "use it or lose it." Any joint or muscle used infrequently will lose part of its function. If there is a lack of movement, we will typically experience mobility as more deliberate, difficult, and stiffer, and accompanied by more pain and discomfort. Simple routine activities such as standing up from a chair, carrying groceries, bending over to tie our shoes, and lifting children or objects can become difficult and cause injury.

Exercise and movement promote all kinds of changes in the brain, including neural growth, reduced inflammation, and new activity patterns that promote feelings of calm and well-being. Additionally, brain sensitivity increases for the hormones serotonin and norepinephrine, relieving feelings of depression. And mood can benefit, no matter the intensity of the physical activity. Conscious breathing, performed during activities such as yoga, can decrease anxiety; 15 minutes of vigorous activity, such as running, or 1 hour of moderate physical activity, such as fast walking, can reduce the risk of major depression by 26%.[3]

According to the American Psychological Association, exercise drives the body's systems to work and communicate more closely (heart with liver with stomach with kidney, etc.). These systems are controlled by our central and autonomic (sympathetic and parasympathetic) nervous systems, which are also communicating with each other: "This workout of the body's communication system may be the true value of exercise; the more sedentary we get, the less efficient our bodies are in responding to stress."[4]

Studies show that regular exercise helps lower levels of cortisol (a stress hormone), improve sleep quality, and reduce stress.[5] Sleep quality is improved by allowing smoother and more regular transitions between the cycles and phases of sleep. Active individuals have fewer episodes of sleeplessness, fall asleep easier, and sleep more soundly than sedentary individuals. Aerobic movement three times a week has been shown to increase the amount of time spent sleeping and decrease pre-sleep anxiety in individuals who suffer from sleeping difficulties. Changes in body temperature, promoted by exercise, trigger areas in the brain that also help initiate sleep.

For so many reasons, therefore, exercise plays a crucial role in making life wonderful. Many of us try to exercise often and don't always succeed; we may succumb to defeat and live with guilt and shame. Guilt and shame can then motivate us to get back to a program, but only out of obligation rather than willingness and enjoyment. Thus, it ends up feeling like more work we have to do, rather than want to do. And, it becomes self-punishing, obsessive, or attached to an outcome (e.g., calorie burning, weight/fat loss, or muscle building).

In fact, forcing ourselves to exercise requires that we suppress our dislike or dread for what we are about to do, and requires some level of mobilization to overcome that dread. This all will be interpreted by the body as a type of threat, in which we have to confront something we don't want to do or else there will be harmful consequences. And we know from earlier chapters that this type of suppression and mobilization shifts our body into a proinflammatory physiological state that is counter to, and likely reverses, some of the anti-inflammatory health benefits we were hoping to stimulate with exercise in the first place.

In other words, don't undo the benefits of activity by forcing yourself to do something that you don't want to do at that moment. Instead of running, consider a leisurely walk or bike ride. Maybe you could meet some friends and shoot hoops or play some soccer? Remember that when you connect to your needs (movement and health), rather than adhere rigidly to a strategy or schedule (running on Monday, lifting on Tuesday), additional options naturally present themselves.

It might be helpful to re-frame exercise as movement throughout our day. Going for a mile walk to strengthen your legs, burn some calories, and stretch your muscles is an example of *exercise*. Walking a mile to the store because you need to pick up something for dinner is an example of *movement*. Both may use the body in the same way, but the intention of the action is significantly different: the former involves carved-out time for movement and the latter involves movement as a part of everyday living.

Move because you love it. Move often, without a rigid structure, and focus on enjoying your chosen activities because it brings you joy to do so and supports your health and well-being.

What motivates your movement?

Our daughter Jordan, age eight, is an example of someone who will not do something if she doesn't find it enjoyable. She hates exercising for the sake of exercising. In fact, when we ask her to join us on a walk, she will refuse. If we say it is great exercise, she won't care and it likely will increase her resistance. However, when we ask her if she wants to go on a "wander" where she walks wherever her body takes her, turning whenever she is moved to do so and exploring whatever she desires along her path, then she is excited. In other words, she is excited to go on an exploration or "wander" but hates going on walks for exercise where we just do a lap or two around the block. She wants to connect with nature and see the flowers and check out the birds; she loves the movement that is required to support that. Our recommendation is to take Jordan's lead and find what motivates your movement and allows you to move with excitement and joy.

We can always do something that feels fun, celebrates our bodies, and is a form of self-expression inspired by self-love and self-care. The options are limited only by your imagination and include ones that readily come to mind as forms of "exercise" such as hiking, biking, walking, running, swimming, yoga, and the gym as well as ones we might not think of in that way such as gardening, dancing, playing with kids, and walking a pet.

In a British study by Biomed Central Public Health, researchers found that a dog owner's daily walk was, on average, 22 minutes longer than walks taken by those without dogs.[6] At 154 minutes per week, even that *extra* time walking is four minutes more than the 150 minutes recommended by the World Health Organization. If you love animals and are able, consider adopting a dog to motivate and inspire you to get outdoors and walk. Instead of thinking you will have to take your new canine for a walk, think of it as your dog taking you out for walks!

A touching video went viral about a middle-aged man who was obese and had developed type 2 diabetes, high cholesterol, and high blood pressure and spent hundreds of dollars on medication every month. He reached his breaking point when he could no longer fit in an airplane seat, and there were no seatbelt extensions big enough. He researched and found a nutritionist who helped him make dietary changes but also instructed him to adopt a shelter dog. The man went to the local shelter and asked for what he thought would be a good match: a middle-aged, overweight dog. The man and the dog, whom he named Peety, immediately connected. Because the dog needed exercise, the man started walking the dog thirty minutes a day. As a result of eating a healthier diet and daily movement, within a year the man lost 140 pounds, reversed his diabetes, lowered his cholesterol, and was taken off his medications by his doctor. Peety lost 25 pounds! The man went on to fulfill his dream of training for and running a marathon. The man said about Peety, "I don't know who saved who."

Owning a pet is just one of many strategies. Did you love playing sports as a kid? Or do you have fond memories of messing around with friends and family at a gathering or in the park where you all played a game without keeping score? Reintroduce that sense of play and try participating in sports with friends, family, or coworkers for fun and without competition, whether it's shooting hoops on the basketball court, tossing a football, kicking a soccer ball, playing volleyball on the beach, playing baseball or softball with the kids, jumping on a trampoline, or taking a no-destination bike ride.

Exercising with others provides an opportunity for increased social contact. Many of us need the motivation of our peers. It helps to have the support and encouragement from others in the same boat, and sharing our struggles and successes enables us to feel less alone. Also, it gives us accountability to the people expecting us to participate. Whenever possible, schedule a walk, a class, or other activity with a friend or colleague. You will be less likely to change your mind if you know someone else is waiting for you and counting on you to be there. Plus, it can be a lot more fun and the time spent will likely feel like it flew by!

Treat your chosen movement as play and do it for fun—purely because you enjoy it and because you CAN.

"One foot in front of the other.
Repeat as often as necessary to finish."
—HARUKI MURAKAMI

Some important statistics[7]

- *1 in 3 children is physically active every day*
- *< 5% of adults are physically active for 30 minutes a day*
- *1 in 3 adults achieve the recommended amount of physical activity each week*
- *≤ 34% of adults ages 65-74 are physically active*
- *≤ 44% of adults 75 years or older are physically active*
- *Children spend > 7 ½ hours in front of a screen daily*
- *Only 6 states require physical education in every grade, K-12 (Illinois, Hawaii, Massachusetts, Mississippi, New York, and Vermont)*

To optimize your health and well-being, vary your movement to incorporate aerobic activity, muscle strengthening, flexibility, and balance.

Aerobic and resistance training

- Studies show that combining aerobic exercise with resistance training can maximize fat loss and muscle mass maintenance, which is essential for maintaining strong bones and keeping off extra weight.
- More than 80% of adults and adolescents do not meet the guidelines for aerobic and muscle-strengthening activities.

Aerobic training recommendations of the American Heart Association for adults 18-65:
- Moderate intensity for a minimum of 30 minutes, five days of the week (≥150min/wk)
- Or vigorous intensity for a minimum of 20 minutes, three days a week (≥75min/wk)

Note: For substantial health benefits, adults should engage in at least 150-300 minutes a week of moderate-intensity aerobic exercise, 75 min-150 min a week of vigorous-intensity aerobic physical activity, or an equivalent combination of moderate- and vigorous-intensity aerobic exercise spread throughout the week.

What you can do aerobically:
- Run, walk, hike, dance, or do housework at a fast pace

Resistance training recommendations of the American Heart Association for adults 18-65:
- Add moderate to high intensity muscle-strengthening activities, a minimum of 2-3 days each week with 2-4 sets per major muscle group.

What can you do for resistance and muscle strengthening:
- weightlifting, yoga, Pilates, walking

Flexibility exercises

- Flexibility protects against injury. Stiff, shorter muscle fibers may not only increase risk of injury but also lead to other issues ranging from back pain to balance problems.[8]
- Flexibility enhances athletic performance. According to Harvard Health, "A well-stretched muscle more easily achieves its full range of motion. This improves athletic performance—imagine an easier, less restricted golf swing or tennis serve—and functional abilities, such as reaching, bending, or stooping during daily tasks."[9]

Flexibility training recommendation of the American College of Sports Medicine and American Heart Association:
- A minimum of 2-3 days per week holding each stretch for 10-30 seconds to mild discomfort (a total of 60 seconds per exercise), 3-4 repetitions per stretch

What you can do for flexibility:
- Stretch all muscle groups. You can use your favorite stretches or find new ones online.
- Experts no longer recommend stretching before exercise. Warm up for 5-10 minutes or wait until finished with the activity and cool down. Repeat each stretch once on each side to stretch each muscle group for approximately 60 seconds. Little by little, extend the duration. Extend the stretch to where you feel mild tension and hold the position without bouncing. Hold the stretch for 30 seconds while breathing in and out calmly.

Balance exercises

- Balance helps reduce falls and related injuries. If not practiced regularly, neural connections are lost and balance deteriorates. Therefore, it is vital to continue balancing activities when healthy and as part of injury recovery programs.
- Good balance requires strong stabilization muscles, including those around the hips, knees, and ankles.
- Good balance requires good posture, so it's essential to include that awareness.

Balance training recommendations of the American Heart Association:
- Exercises can be done daily and as often as you enjoy
- ≥ 3 days per week for older adults, especially those at risk for falls

What you can do for balance:
- Incorporate balance into daily life. Stand on one leg whenever you're waiting in line at the theater, bank, or grocery store. Or try it when brushing your teeth by spending one minute on one leg while brushing the upper teeth and another minute on the other while brushing the lower teeth.
- Keep a wobble board in your office. Stand on it during a break or whenever you're on the phone.

- Practice sitting down and getting up from a chair without using your hands.
- Combined balance and step training (CBST) routines provide benefits in both balance and mobility. These activities include walking backward and sideways, walking on a plank, stepping on and off curbs, practicing heel and toe raises, and catching a ball while standing on an unstable surface. The goal is to stabilize the body under increasingly difficult circumstances. Start by balancing on a flat surface, then on an unstable surface, then on an uneven surface while someone pushes you or throws a ball.
- Practice walking heel to toe like a tightrope walker, placing the heel of one foot directly in front of the toes of the opposite foot each time you take a step.
- Increase the difficulty of your practice. For example:
  - Stand on one leg for 30 seconds and then repeat with the other leg (use the wall for stabilization if needed).
  - Once able to do that without holding on to anything, try it with your eyes closed.
  - Once able to do that without holding on to anything, try it with a wobble board or something similar.
  - Once able to do that without holding on to anything, try it on tiptoes. You can bend over while balancing and lifting the other leg in the air or behind you.

CHAPTER 10

Play

Pillar 4

"We don't stop playing because we grow old;
we grow old because we stop playing."

—GEORGE BERNARD SHAW

WHAT DID YOU LOVE TO do as a child that excited you? Was it simply goofing off and joking around with friends? Throwing a frisbee? Listening to records and playing air guitar? Dive bombing into a swimming pool or lake? Sword fighting with sticks? Dancing, playing charades, and riding bikes with your friends? When did you stop playing, and why?

In the blockbuster movie "Big," starring Tom Hanks, a thirteen-year-old boy named Josh finds "Zoltar Speaks," a magical wish-fulfilling game, at a traveling carnival. Frustrated because a girl he likes witnesses him getting rejected from a ride for not being tall enough, Josh puts a coin in the slot and says, "I wish I were big." He wakes up the next day in a man's body, but inside he is still a boy, so he continues acting like one. He is silly, spontaneous, loves games, joking, riding his bike, and jumping on a trampoline.

Josh gets a computer job with a toy manufacturer. At a famous New York City toy store, the toy maker's CEO spots Josh playing with uninhibited exuberance. The next day, Josh gets promoted to his dream job, testing (playing with) new toys. Because of his playfulness and fearless creativity, Josh quickly gets promoted again and rises in the corporate ranks. Suddenly, he has meetings, deadlines, and responsibilities. It's all work and no play. His adult life is now full of expectations, worry, and stress. In that stressful environment focused on accomplishing tasks and goals, he quickly loses the joy and enthusiasm that differentiated him from all the other executives and made him so attractive to the leadership. Downtrodden, Josh laments, "I am going to be thirty years old for the rest of my life." Luckily, Josh tracks down Zoltar, who grants his wish to turn back into a boy. Josh and his best friend are back on their bikes, singing, clowning around, and playing.

"We are a nation of exhausted and overstressed adults," notes author, speaker, and psychologist Brené Brown in her book, *The Gifts of Imperfection.* "Exhaustion and productivity become badges of honor."[1]

Adults are taught to pursue a trade or career and work hard until we retire or die. We judge play as a guilty pleasure: unproductive, impractical, and an impediment to reaching our goal of earning money to provide food and necessities, among other things.

But play is as essential a need as food, water, sleep, and sex. It's a biological drive that plays a crucial role in our well-being. As children play, they learn how to relate to other children in social situations. They consciously and subconsciously read a variety of social cues from other kids, perfecting their ability to discern safety from danger.

In other words, play with other people is essential for teaching our nervous system how to regulate and switch from survival mode to safety/pro-social mode. Without "practicing" play, we can easily perceive safe situations as dangerous, leading to the stimulation of our threat physiology and the resulting proinflammatory state. As adults, we can use play to allow our physiology to take a rest from being productive, effective, or vigilant. We cannot connect when we are in survival mode, so we can use play to shut off survival mode, shift into a state of safety, and enjoy connection. In addition, play is one way to give our nervous system a physiological break from hypervigilance—not to mention, it's just fun and pleasurable. So why do we neglect play when we grow up? And what is the cost?

Once mammals are safe, rested, and satiated, it's natural for them to play. Animals with the highest survival rates spend time playing, eating, sleeping, and mating. But if we feel we are in danger (perceived or real), our drive for play will be halted. In non-human mammals, the threat comes from a predator or dangerous weather. For humans, that threat is usually the stress and worry we create by living in survival mode in an effort to meet the needs of our family, friends, and work.

Neglecting time for play may feel convenient in the short term, especially when we view our other responsibilities as more essential to survival. But if we neglect it for long periods, it undeniably affects our health and happiness.

Our adult brains aren't developing as much as those of children, so the drive for play is lower and more easily dismissed. But human brains are malleable and can continue developing and growing for our entire lives. Play assists and, some argue, stimulates this neurogenesis in adults, as it does in children.

There is evidence showing that rats raised in enriched environments are smarter, with larger brains and more developed cortexes. One of the keys to enriching their environments is providing a variety of toy-like objects and socialization opportunities for play with other rats. It turns out that rats that play have better brain development.[2]

Play does not demand a rigid way of doing things; it's improvisational; it keeps us open to chance and change. Play provides a space for new insight and creativity. When we try new behaviors and act outside of our "normal," we stumble onto new strategies for life, from new movements and behaviors to new thoughts and ways of being. Animals that grow out of play transition into a state of rigidity and fixed behaviors. They, like us, stop developing. When we lose interest in new and different things, we decrease opportunities to experience pleasure in our external world. In short, when we stop playing, we start dying.

According to Stuart Brown, MD, author of the best-selling book *Play: How it Shapes the Brain, Opens the Imagination, and Invigorates the Soul,* play deprivation is rampant and harmful: "What you begin to see when there's major play deprivation in an otherwise competent adult is that they're not much fun to be around… You begin to see that the perseverance and joy in work are lessened, and that life is much more laborious."[3]

Play deprivation has huge costs[4]

· Emotional dysregulation
· Greater prevalence of depression and addiction
· Increased rigidity and inflexibility
· Decreased adaptability and self-regulation
· Diminished impulse control and anger management
· Superficial interpersonal relationships

"Play is something done for its own sake… It's voluntary, it's pleasurable, it offers a sense of engagement, it takes you out of time. And the act itself is more important than the outcome," says Brown.[5] "Play is an activity that is content-free, purposeless, all-consuming, and fun without a need to accomplish any required goals or tasks." When we are engaged in play, we enter a flow state and are not focused on the self, on how we look, feel, or think. Instead, we are absorbed in the activity and free from the constrictions of time. This pleasure drives our desire, and the joy of play urges us to keep doing it. We often don't want it to end, and when it does, we often want to do it again. Play's inherent attraction is that it's fun and feels good. There's no opportunity to get bored. Play is pure freedom; you don't need to be practical, please others, be responsible or efficient, or feel guilt and worry.

Sadly, Americans spend most of their leisure time on devices, which include watching television. Television, not a form of play as we define it, accounts for three hours a day in contrast to about eighteen minutes of participating in sports, exercise, and recreation.[6]

Only one in five adults participates in recreational activities daily. With children, there is a deficit of play in their daily routines, as schools replace play with more didactics. Pediatricians now actively recommend play as an essential component of brain development and overall health. Brown adamantly claims, "The science is clear: The joy of play nourishes our minds like food nourishes our bodies."

"A child who does not play is not a child."
—PABLO NERUDA

One survey of 68 kindergartens determined that about half of kindergartens surveyed engaged in free play, far less than the amount recommended by the Early Childhood Environment Rating Scale-Revised (ECERS-R).[7]

About 40 million children (55% of children 3-4 years old) globally have fathers "who do not play or engage in early learning activities with them," according to a UNICEF analysis.[8]

We must safeguard time to play the same way we protect time to eat and sleep. It's not something you do only when you have finished everything else—we know that time will never come! Instead, be intentional, make room for play on your schedule, and protect that time just like you would a meeting or important call. If that sounds challenging to you, then take some time to reflect on why that is the case. Do you not value play? Do you value other areas more than play? Do you not really know how to play anymore?

Play, like singing or running, is a skill that needs honing. Everyone knows how to do it, but you can be much better at it with practice. It is normal to lose proficiency in play if you haven't done it in a while, so don't let that initial awkwardness or discomfort dissuade you from re-engaging with this essential part of life. We can all add play to our calendars and would benefit greatly by supporting a world that values play as much as it does productivity.

Sadly, this approach disrupts conventional establishments where it is believed that making time for play jeopardizes work. But play can be adapted to any environment. And contrary to the traditional view of the workplace, it provides benefits even at work. According to an article published by the Association for Psychological Science: "Research has found evidence that play at work is linked with less fatigue, boredom, stress, and burnout in individual workers. Play is also positively associated with job satisfaction, a sense of competence, and creativity. Studies show that when a participant receives a task that is presented playfully, they are more involved and spend more time on the task."[9]

Work and play are two sides of the same coin, and we don't need to play all day to fulfill our needs. In reality, even a little play in our routine can make us more productive and joyful. Long work hours make us *appear* more productive but don't increase output or inspire our best results.

At WeHeal, our workplace culture incorporates a focus on connection and play. We prioritize time for regular connection and play. For example, we regularly make time to joke and laugh, check in on each other's lives, and celebrate life events and experiences with each other. What we have found is that our team finds this approach restoring and inspiring. This has translated into greater efficiency and productivity for both individuals and the company overall. In other words, don't be penny wise and dollar foolish when it comes to incorporating play into your team.

Play fosters trust, creative meeting climates, bonding, social interaction, and a sense of solidarity in work environments. It also decreases boundaries between hierarchical roles. Play cultivates a friendly atmosphere, a high commitment culture, ability to relate to an unknown future, and flexible organizational decision-making. Play helps you recover from the stress of the day and gives your subconscious mind space to keep working. By equally prioritizing play, you become more efficient and productive at work.

Play has equal benefits in your personal life.

- **Brain Health:** Play evolved over centuries and helps sculpt and maintain brain health. In the words of Stuart Brown, "...play seems to be one of the most advanced methods that nature has invented to allow a complex brain to create itself."[10] Lack of play causes a decrease in brain and muscle fiber development, communication, problem-solving, and social skills. In contrast, play affects the health of the frontal cortex, where cognition and executive functions (discernment of information, organization of thought and feeling, addressing the future) live. It helps the brain learn and adapt through simulation and testing, making new connections, and innovating. Play is the canvas on which we can create new combinations, using cognition and imagination to see what works and doesn't. In fact, play, along with REM sleep, seem to work hand-in-hand with brain development and neural evolution. REM sleep tests and strengthens neural connections, while play creates new connections that didn't exist before (safely testing these new circuits during play when "survival" is not at stake).

In nature, play is how the young practice their survival and reproductive skills. Additionally, research shows[11] that active play stimulates nerve growth in an area of the brain called the amygdala, where we integrate and regulate emotions. This is particularly important in processing danger and threat and generating messages of safety. Play is actually essential to practicing learning how to mobilize and then come back to safety. Sometimes we get too aggressive or overreact during play, but when this happens, we can easily recover as well as learn and fine-tune our reactivity—lessons that we can apply, consciously or not, in life.

Exposure can be health-promoting. For example, being exposed to germs can help fine-tune our immune system, whereas being in an overly sterile environment can increase our chances of creating hyper-reactive immune systems, as is seen with autoimmune diseases. Similarly, exposure to conflict is essential to fine-tuning our emotional reactivity. Children who have not had the opportunity to experience conflict (being kept safe and never exposed to challenge and danger) are less resilient when dealing with discomfort and have a decreased ability to navigate obstacles and persevere in a socially connected way. Whether it is with play, germs, or social conflict, the absence of practice and exposure leads to a state of hypersensitivity as well as physical and/or emotional reactivity. Play allows us to learn, in a safe environment, how to navigate the complicated social world in which we live.

Play has also been shown to help protect people from dementia. Engaging in leisure activities such as playing board games, reading, playing a musical instrument, and dancing are associated with a reduced risk of dementia.[12]

- Play **improves mood and reduces anxiety**
  Play has a bidirectional connection with the autonomic nervous systems. You can't be anxious when playing; you can't play when perceiving a threat. Play is one of our most powerful tools to send messages of safety signals to the brain. In fact, the American Academy of Pediatrics links increases in depression and anxiety to a lack of unstructured playtime. Neglecting play causes our mood to suffer with decreased optimism, anhedonia (inability to feel pleasure), and the failure to sustain pleasurable feelings. In contrast, play enhances self-regulation, empathy, and group management skills, in addition to reducing stress and releasing feel-good happy hormones (endorphins, dopamine, and serotonin).[13]

Cheering an entrance

One of our family's favorite ways to play, which also increases connection, is cheering an entrance. When someone comes in the door we will randomly cheer really loudly, chant their name, hoot and holler, jump up and down, and do whatever else we can to show our excitement. It is simple, fun, and extremely connecting. What's more, it is therapeutic. Don't take our word for it, try it out with your family!

Matt's story

I remember a time when I was walking in the house after a long day of things not going as planned. I was feeling irritable and angry with a bit of head tension. Independently (unaware of my state), Alona and Kylee gave me a cheer upon entry that made me smile. My response was to start cheering with them. Jordan,

---

who arrived shortly after me, heard the cheering and ran in to see what was going on. As she entered, the three of us began to cheer for her. The huge smile on her face had us all smiling as we cheered her name while clapping and jumping up and down. My mood was immediately shifted and the tension in my head was gone. I was so pleasantly surprised to notice what a shift this simple intervention had on my body and mood.

- Play **modifies inflammation**

During play, we tend to laugh more. Laughter can influence levels of inflammatory cytokine levels and release natural pain-killers, reducing inflammation and pain in the body. It can also decrease blood pressure, enhance circulation, help muscles relax, and improve your immune system. The famous Dr. Patch Adams knew this when he created the Gesundheit! Institute in 1971. He spent his career teaching medical students to cultivate connection with their patients. His prescription for care relied on humor and play, which he saw as essential to physical and emotional health.

- Play **helps manage weight and contributes to overall well-being**

Physical activity and free play are essential to maintaining a healthy weight and supporting cognitive, physical, social, and emotional development and well-being. As children, many of us didn't worry about our weight. Instead, we rode our bikes outside, played catch and hide and seek, and ran around with our friends having fun. We were never bored, and we didn't mindlessly snack. Instead, our parents called us in from outside and scolded us for being late for dinner!

The decline in children's active play is worrying to say the least. In one study looking at children aged 10-16, they found that children spent 75.5% of the day inactive with an average of 10.4 waking hours each day relatively motionless. What's more, they spent only 12.6 minutes per day in vigorous physical activity! As we already know, a sedentary lifestyle often goes hand in hand with obesity and other health problems, but this study demonstrated that "increased high-level physical activity is an important component in the development of self-esteem in children."[14]

- Play **contributes to intellectual and creative growth**
  Play improves intelligence, adaptability, joy, social relationships, empathy, creativity, innovation, mental health, self-regulation, curiosity, perseverance, optimism, and progressive mastery.

- Play **enhances connection and strengthens relationships**
  Play helps maintain social well-being when gathering and solidifying teams, connects people, and helps build community. Play also keeps relationships and partnerships healthy and builds closeness with those you love. Dr. Stuart Brown says, "The couples who sustain a sense of mutual playfulness with each other tend to work out the wrinkles in their relationships much better than those who are really serious."[15]

Understanding that we need more play is one thing; making it happen is entirely another. This is largely because we are not very good at identifying how badly we are doing without play, erroneously assuming that however we currently feel is the "normal" way to feel. Therefore, we underestimate the impact lack of play has on our lives. Play is natural, despite it not feeling so. We must find our way back to it, just like Josh in "Big." Initially, you may need to try something that feels unnatural only because it is not yet habitual (more on that in Chapter 14). As a result, to incorporate more play requires intention, first and foremost. Here are some ideas and strategies that might be helpful as you aim to incorporate more play in your daily life:

1) Take a play history to determine your "play personality." (See sidebar on Play Personality.) Notice what you were naturally drawn to as a child and see what resonates now. Allow yourself to identify, without judgment, the things you loved as a child.

Think of something you enjoyed so much that you got lost in it, time and time again. Notice how you feel when you imagine playing in similar ways. For example, did you love horseback riding? Imagine horseback riding now. Or dancing as a child? Imagine dancing similarly now. Were you more of an outdoors type or did you prefer playing inside? Did you like groups or solo play?

Some of us are inclined to engage in physical play such as gymnastics, martial arts, jumping on a trampoline, riding a bike, roller skating, skateboarding, jumping rope, frisbee, swimming, and dancing. And for others, play is a form of art such as photography, painting, drawing, molding clay, singing, playing guitar, piano, or other instruments. What did you love to do and never wanted to stop?

Play can also include things we enjoy, such as cooking and exercise. But it is play only as long as we do it with joy and without the pressure to show results or reach a goal. When you cook, do it for fun, creating a spontaneous meal because you love cooking, not due to the pressure of a dinner party. Or jump rope and shoot hoops because it's fun and takes your mind off your responsibilities, not because you want to lose weight or win a game.

2) To help make play a habit, develop a small ritual (or rituals) that you want to incorporate into your daily life. You can include rituals in already planned activities or block separate time in your daily schedule. Start small, so you don't feel overwhelmed trying to "fit it in." For example, crank up the music and dance while doing the dishes or cleaning the house. Make folding laundry a family race and see who finishes first. Take five minutes before dinner to dance, an hour a week to shoot hoops with a friend, or go golfing on a weekend day. The opportunities are abundant if you make some space and time for them.

3) Keep a journal. Often, when we are in the moment, we aren't aware of the pleasant feelings that arise during play, so we don't appreciate the full value of it. Think back to the play activity

performed, even if just for a few minutes. As you reflect, note the sensations you feel in your body and heart and write them down. Take turns sharing what you notice with loved ones, if you are comfortable doing so. It is helpful to refer to your journal on occasion to remind you of the personal benefits you derive from play.

Matt's story—dancing like nobody was watching

After a long day of working hard at my desk, I was rewarded with a headache and exhaustion. I thought I needed rest and that lying on the couch watching TV might help restore some of my energy. What I realized after a while was that I wasn't really tired and this strategy was not working. Remembering polyvagal theory and threat physiology, I realized that working with the intensity I had, desiring to be as efficient and productive as possible, was leading me to be in a chronic state of threat or high alert and survival mode. In my body and mind, it was as if a bomb was under my desk about to go off if I didn't get everything done.

What we know from polyvagal theory is that after sustained periods of being mobilized in response to a perceived threat (in this case deadlines, back-to-back phone calls, reports to read, content to create, people to serve), eventually the body will shut down because it cannot remain mobilized indefinitely. When mobilization (fight/flight) does not neutralize the threat, the body starts to shut down or immobilize (freeze/faint) to preserve resources.

I realized that what I thought was fatigue was actually a shift to this immobilized state. That meant that resting on the couch wouldn't fix the problem, as my body was not in need of rest. What my body really needed was safety, to shift out of relating to the world as a threat and into seeing the world as a safe place. One of the best ways to help your nervous system shift into a state of safety is to connect and play. Remember that our nervous system is bidirectional or "works both ways" so we can feel safe and as a result then be open to play—OR we can play and then as a result of that play start to feel safe inside. Knowing that, I decided to turn on some music and dance with my kids. Initially, my body resisted this intention because it mistakenly believed I was tired. Persevering, I continued to dance to a fun, upbeat song with a big smile on my face, as I sang (horribly) along. My daughters were smiling and we were making eye contact and laughing; they love to sing and dance together.

We danced like nobody was watching, which is important because dancing where you are self-conscious will actually shift you back towards threat physiology (wanting to dance in an acceptable way). Bringing children or friends into this is very helpful, as it stacks the deck towards safety by dancing together (connection), to fun music (sounds of safety), with big smiles (visual cues of safety), singing or humming (triggers nerves in larynx towards safety), and being as silly as you can (play). When I smile, laugh, sing, dance, and do whatever I can to trigger the "play reflex," I can see how quickly my headache and sense of tiredness resolve. In other words, I shift out of immobilization and back towards a pro-social sense of safety. Given that sitting at your desk for eight hours isn't physically exhausting, why would your body be physically tired? It is helpful to realize that the heavy, weighted feeling you have associated with a need to lay on the couch is really a need to shift into a state of safety.

After I got over the initial resistance hump telling me to lay on the couch, my exhausted feeling dissipated and I ended up glad that I had chosen to play instead. Try it yourself using your preferred method of play and fun, as that is the key to helping you most quickly and efficiently shift into a state of safety and connection.

"Plan the play, then play the plan, you can do it,
everyone can!… What are we gonna play today?"
—THE MUPPETS OF SESAME STREET

What play personality are you?

According to Stuart Brown, most people have a dominant mode of play. By identifying your type or types amongst the eight different options, you increase awareness of what you most enjoy, making it easier to bring more play into your life.

Identify your play personality. Do you have a single type? Do you have a main type with other subtypes? Use this to help direct your attention to areas that could better meet your need for play.

The Joker

Loves to make people laugh, tell jokes, or do impressions. Known as the class clown. Gains social acceptance by making others laugh.
Play opportunities: tell jokes, watch comedy, and be silly.

Kinesthetic

Loves movement and prefers movement in order to think and be most successful. For example, a child may struggle with reading until allowed to bounce on a ball and read at the same time.
Play opportunities: yoga, hiking, sports, running, dance, swimming, and jumping rope. Learn or play whatever sport or activity you enjoy.

Explorer

Loves to play through discovery and exploration that can be physical (travel to new places), mental (discover new subjects and viewpoints), or emotional (experiencing new or deeper feelings).

Play opportunities: see new places, learn more about an area you enjoy, use arts to experience emotion, go on adventures, research your curiosities, pursue your fascinations, listen to new music, and meet new people.

Competitor

Loves to win and set records alone or with a team, loves to keep score and be number one in games with others or alone.
Play opportunities: play games, pursue goals you set, facilitate office competitions, and watch competitive sports.

Director

Loves to organize and execute events and provide experiences for their family, friends, and community.
Play opportunities: host social events, organize, plan, and lead groups.

Collector

Loves to have and organize the most interesting collections (artifacts, experiences, or whatever interests them). Collectors will want to methodically collect all they can and organize the "evidence" of their collection.
Play opportunities: Collect what you enjoy and show off your collections. Explore and discover new stuff/experiences to add to their collections (differs from Explorer who does it for the experience).

Artist/Creator

Loves anything creative and artistic (examples: painting, drawing, building, sewing, gardening, playing music, singing, and fixing), and enjoys making things (whether functional, silly, practical, or beautiful).
Play opportunities: creating art or making new things, discovering art, sharing creations and art with others. Find the art

or artistic/creative activities you enjoy, share your creations/art with others, take time to observe your creations/art, and make and/or develop things.

Storyteller

Loves imagination and experiencing a story in some way. They love the drama around the activity but don't need to win or create it.

Play opportunities: Do anything around a story (write, tell, listen, read, and watch), be part of the story such as with performing arts, go to the theater, movies, and other performances.

CHAPTER 11

Sleep

Pillar 5

"The best bridge between despair and
hope is a good night's sleep."

—E. JOSEPH COSSMAN

I'LL SLEEP WHEN I'M DEAD. *Sleep is a luxury I cannot afford. I'd rather be tired than broke.* These are just a few of the modern-day mantras of a sleep-deprived world in which productivity reigns supreme. The irony is that in our quest for productivity, we sacrifice the one thing that favorably impacts it the most: sleep.

Simply put, we need a good night's sleep to function during the day. Believe it or not, the brain is nearly as metabolically active when asleep as it is when awake. It is busy performing many essential functions, including detoxification and integration of information to support learning and memory, that cannot occur throughout the day and that need sufficient time to be completed while we are sleeping.

Sleep triggers a soothing effect on our nervous system, sending calming signals that reduce the damage of physiological stress on the body. Sleep recalibrates our emotional brain circuits, allowing us to navigate social and psychological challenges. Proper sleep repairs and restocks the immune system, helping us fight malignancy, prevent infection, and avoid other threats of sickness. Sleep influences our alertness, memory, mood, and social and emotional intelligence.

The less you sleep, the worse your concentration and the more difficulty you have with focusing. Logical reasoning and complex thought become impaired, and confusion can ensue. Sleep deprivation affects our performance, decreases our output, and ultimately deteriorates our personal and professional relationships. It is hard to optimize our internal world without adequate sleep, and it's hard to connect and contribute to others with joy if we are tired due to lack of sleep. What's more, we are more likely to perceive an innocuous communication from someone as threatening or take it personally when we are tired. We may run out of patience with our children or hear unintended criticism in our partner's words when we would not have if we were well rested. By choosing to get less sleep, you unfortunately also choose to increase disconnection with others, especially those closest to you.

The two main categories of sleep
REM = Rapid Eye Movement sleep
NREM sleep = Non-Rapid Eye Movement sleep

We go through 90-minute cycles involving both NREM sleep and REM sleep throughout the night, with more NREM sleep occurring early in the night, and more of our REM sleep occurring later as morning approaches. As a result, if you wake up after six hours instead of getting a total of eight hours, you may have cut your sleep by 25% but could be cutting out 50% of your total very important REM sleep. There is no way to "hack" sleep; regardless of what time you go to bed or wake up, if you try going to bed later you lose a disproportionate amount of NREM sleep; and if you try waking up after a suboptimal amount of sleep, you will lose a disproportionate amount of REM sleep. If people knew even 10% of what we teach about sleep, then they would prioritize and protect their entire sleep window and never again trade it for more time in their day!

NREM sleep and REM sleep work together to tend to the day's new inputs, sorting new and old information and determining what to store and discard. NREM sleep eliminates, weeds out, and removes unnecessary neural connections, while REM sleep strengthens remaining connections by integrating, interconnecting, adding detail, and blending. Imagine it this way: NREM sleep prunes unnecessary plants in our garden while REM sleep tends to those we want to keep and helps them grow. Together, they tend to our ability to learn, consolidate our recollections of experiences into long-term memories, and integrate logic and emotion to best navigate our interpersonal world and its related challenges. In this manner, we heal painful experiences and traumatic memories, integrate knowledge, create new solutions and ideas, and call upon our past to address current and future problems.

There are many scientific studies about why and how we sleep, and the data concur: humans need roughly eight hours of solid sleep per night for our bodies and brains to rest and repair. But instead of getting the necessary amount of shut-eye, we use stimulant drugs, over-the-counter pills, and caffeinated energy drinks to stay awake and power through our day. The demand is high, with about 90% of people on the planet using caffeine. This includes children consuming soda.[1] Is it any wonder that there's a coffee shop on almost every corner of the developed world?

Most coffee-drinkers don't realize that when we ingest caffeine at noon, a quarter of it is still circulating in our bloodstream at midnight. Caffeine blocks the receptor site for adenosine, a neuromodulator in our body that causes sleepiness. Adenosine builds up during the day (called sleep pressure), so we can fall and stay asleep at night. When we consume caffeine, adenosine absorption is blocked and the adenosine has no place to go. When the caffeine finally wears off, the adenosine build-up suddenly floods the receptors and causes us to crash, making us even more sleepy than before we had that cup of joe. To wake from this somnolence, we consume more caffeine, perpetuating the cycle. Essentially, we need caffeine to help us recover from the effects of caffeine. This lingering caffeine in our bodies adversely affects deep sleep. Even if that afternoon cup of coffee or tea doesn't prevent us from falling asleep, it affects the overall quality of our sleep. And with impaired sleep, many metabolic functions in the body and brain are adversely affected.

For our early ancestors, the hunter-gatherer cultures, sleep cycles were dictated by the earth's rotation around the sun. There was no choice but to sleep just after sunset and wake up at sunrise. Midnight meant the middle of the night or middle point of the solar cycle. Before the advent of artificial light, humans experienced biphasic sleep; we slept when the sun went down, rose with the sunrise, and napped in the afternoon's heat. If sleep was disrupted, it was due to an immediate threat to one's safety, as might arise from a prowling saber-toothed tiger, a bear, or threatening weather.

In the presence of interrupted sleep, our bodies enter survival mode ready to fight the presumed threat. This automatic response to the absence of adequate or appropriate sleep makes sense, given that historically this happened only if there was a physical threat preventing sleep. However, today our bodies still assume there must be some sort of threat present if our sleep gets interrupted or restricted. As such, a lack of sleep (for whatever reason, or no good reason at all) puts our bodies into the same state of threat or high alert or survival mode. Remember that when we are in survival mode, we are in a proinflammatory state, which is appropriate to address tissue damage and other related issues that are temporary in nature. However, when we are in a chronic proinflammatory state, as we are when we regularly under-sleep, disease starts to set in.

Normal is no longer natural

After Thomas Edison created the lightbulb, humans could control our environment and alter the twenty-four-hour cycle of light and dark. Essentially, humans now can decide when it is night and day. While artificial light is one of the significant advances of humankind, it also has its costs. We no longer sleep in that biphasic sleep pattern, but are now mainly monophasic sleepers, meaning we sleep in one long bout. Most people sleep seven hours or less at night, without napping during the day. Midnight is no longer the middle of the night, but instead when many of us fire up our laptops or binge-watch a television series.

Our bodies release a sleep hormone, melatonin, which increases after dark and decreases as morning approaches. When darkness arrives, melatonin signals to the body that it's time to sleep. But the artificial light from our laptops, cell phones, televisions, and certain types of light bulbs can put a brake on the release of melatonin, faking our bodies and brains into staying awake and causing inadequate sleep.

We are the only species to purposefully deprive itself of rest. No animal other than humans consciously robs itself of sleep. As a result, we trudge along during the day, thinking we are functioning at our baseline and not realizing how far below that level we are. We are terrible at noticing how poorly we are doing and how it affects the people around us.

There are still tribes in other parts of the world whose way of life has not changed much over the past thousands of years and who still sleep in a biphasic pattern based on the sun's rising and setting. And in parts of Europe and Mediterranean countries, you will find entire cities shut down in the afternoon for siesta or afternoon nap time. Long-term productivity has not suffered because they have broken up their day with rest. It's a way of life, and in addition to naps, a healthy diet and connection with the community result in happier and healthier populations.

That afternoon dip we feel after lunch continues to be a biological response alerting our bodies to rest. Sadly, the modern world is largely moving away from the traditions of closing shops at noon or taking siestas. Asking your boss for time to take a nap could lose you respect and quite possibly your job. Our regular sleep disruption is no longer due to immediate threats but rather comes from such self-inflicted contrivances as caffeine, stress, and worry. As a result, in areas with previously thriving health, there has been a rise in heart disease and other chronic illnesses, as well as shorter life spans. This is primarily because our bodies don't distinguish between the tiger on the prowl, coffee after lunch, or pressure at the office. Our fight-or-flight response becomes unconsciously routine, taking a toll on our bodies and minds. We routinely trigger the physiological state of threat or high alert that stimulates a proinflammatory cascade, resulting in disease.

Sleep deprivation causes lots of problems

Sleep deprivation leads to increased mortality, 5x more depression, 2x more medical visits and hospitalizations, 4x more accidents, troubles with the family or at work and school, and a decreased quality of life.[2]

Detrimental consequences of sleep deprivation:

- Sleep deficiency is associated with disease in nearly every organ system of our bodies and is linked to seven of the fifteen leading causes of death in the U.S., including cardiovascular disease (heart attacks, vascular stiffness, blockage, stroke, and heart failure), diabetes and insulin resistance, septicemia (infection), cancer, and accidents.[3]
- Poor sleep triggers a threat response, revving the sympathetic "fight-or-flight system" and thereby releasing inflammatory chemicals called cytokines and cortisol that result in increased heart rate, constricted blood vessels, and high blood pressure.
- Loss of sleep may play a key role in activating brain regions that contribute to excessive worrying. The mechanisms involved are thought to mimic the exact ones that make us sensitive to anxiety in areas of the brain that support emotional processing, regulation, and calm. In fact, scientists have found that sleep deprivation and insomnia increase the risk of developing anxiety disorders, a problem that compounds itself because "70-80% of people with clinical anxiety have trouble either falling or staying asleep."[4] Additionally, incessant poor sleep leads to anticipatory anxiety about falling asleep in the future, leading to further trouble sleeping and insufficient quality sleep. It's a vicious and dangerous cycle that also contributes to other mental health concerns including depression and suicidality.

- Inadequate sleep increases our risk of obesity by increasing ghrelin, a hormone that makes us feel hungry, while at the same time suppressing leptin, a complementary hormone that signals satiety. This hormone upheaval results in our feeling hungry and continuing to eat even when our body is full and doesn't need more food. Studies show that sleep-deprived individuals (with sleep deficits of several hours per night) crave about 30-40% more sweets, processed carbs, and salty snacks.[5] Furthermore, the fight-or-flight survival mode from lack of sufficient sleep causes the somnolent person to choose more calorie-dense foods, increases the struggle with impulse control, leads to feeling less satisfied with meals and, as a result, increases overall calorie consumption.

Sleep deprivation affects how you eat

Leptin, the "I'm full" signal, decreases
Ghrelin, the "I'm hungry" signal, increases
Endocannabinoids, the "munchies" signal, increase

- Sleep deprivation impairs the absorption of food and nutrients and can cause gastrointestinal problems including acid reflux, irritable bowel syndrome, abdominal pain and discomfort, nausea, diarrhea, and constipation. In contrast, adequate sleep makes our gut happier because it balances the autonomic nervous system by calming the sympathetic branch. According to polyvagal theory, your stomach and intestines require a steady stream of "you are safe" messaging to flow from the vagus nerve to your viscera for the gut to function normally. When we are in survival/threat mode, the "you are safe" messaging gets turned off in preparation for shifting resources to the areas of the body needed to optimize threat survival. Interrupted and/or reduced sleep is just one of the many ways the "you are safe" message to your gut gets turned off. Therefore, a good night's sleep improves all functioning of our gut, including the health of our microbiome (healthy gut flora), and enhances our metabolism.

- Lack of sleep increases the risk of Alzheimer's disease, immune system impairment (increased risk of getting sick and decreased ability to recover quickly), and reproductive health problems (including reduced testosterone in men and difficulty with conception in women).

- Much like alcohol, sleepiness impairs judgment and results in missed cues, so we don't necessarily know how impaired we are. The consequences of sleep deprivation include increased accidents and errors. Staying awake for seventeen to nineteen hours straight (or only getting six to seven hours of sleep) impacts performance more than a blood-alcohol level of .05 percent. This level of impairment slows an individual's reaction time by about 50% compared to someone who is well-rested. Twenty-four hours of continuous wakefulness impairs performance to a degree comparable to a blood-alcohol level of 0.10 percent, beyond the legal limit for alcohol intoxication in the United States. Based on the best available research, the Institute of Medicine estimates that drowsy driving is responsible for 20% of all motor vehicle crashes. That means that drowsy driving causes 1 million crashes, 500,000 injuries, and 8,000 deaths yearly in the U.S. Is that really worth being able to get a little more done?

Sleep deprivation increases car accidents

⅓ of all adult drivers have fallen asleep at the wheel

* *According to a National Highway Traffic Safety Administration (NHTSA) report, one-third of all adult drivers say they have fallen asleep at the wheel.[6]*

At this point, you may be wondering what an ideal night of sleep even looks like. Think about quantity, efficiency (percentage of time spent asleep), and latency (the time it takes to fall asleep). Ideally, aim for a protected eight-hour sleep window with fifteen to thirty minutes built in beforehand for the time it takes to fall asleep. Protect a ninety-minute window to wind down before getting into bed. Shut off electronics, avoid stress, and connect with others by talking, journaling, or reading a book. Avoid the blue light from electronics just before bed, as it fools the brain into thinking it's still daytime (remember our discussion about melatonin).

It's necessary to monitor our time asleep versus total time in bed. Suppose we get into bed at 10 pm and read for an hour. In that case, our sleep latency period starts at 11 pm, and we count the number of hours of sleep beginning at 11:30 pm.

If you are awake in bed for more than twenty minutes or feeling anxious or worried, get up and do some relaxing activity until you feel sleepy. Ironically, the anxiety from not falling asleep can make it harder to fall asleep. A relaxing activity can include reading, music, a warm bath, or meditation, among others. Although tempting, do not go back to your devices, as this will only impede your sleep even more.

Sample schedule for optimal sleep window

9 – 10:30 pm—90-minute wind down

10:30 – 11 pm—30-minute sleep latency window

11 pm – 7 am—8-hour sleep window

7 – 8 am—If possible, include a 60-minute reentry in the morning with natural light exposure and without focusing on productivity. It's a good time to journal, connect, inspire, imagine, create, move outside, and avoid technology.

Sleep deprivation is rampant

1 in 3 U.S. adults reports they get less than 7 hours of sleep, whereas the ideal amount is closer to 8 hours.[7]

With so many of us experiencing sleep deprivation, the natural next question is, what can we do to enhance our sleep?

- Maintain consistency. The most important rule is to stick to a sleep schedule. Go to sleep and wake up at the same time each day. If you set an alarm, do so for going to and getting up from bed, to prioritize and help set your routine.
- Make time to wind down. Don't overschedule your day and leave yourself without adequate time for unwinding. If you are stressed from the day, living in threat mode, you will have a hard time turning that stress off all of a sudden when it is time to sleep. It is essential that you build opportunities to experience a sense of safety and inner peace throughout your day. When you are unable to regulate and calm yourself before bed, your brain will signal danger and struggle to sleep (like trying to sleep well when a tiger is in the room). This cycle continues because insufficient sleep results in the body remaining stuck in a fight-or-flight, survival, state. So, stress will beget lack of sleep, inducing more stress and further sleep deprivation. One way to decrease evening stress is to avoid stressful activities before bed. This includes checking work emails, watching violent movies, reading violent or stimulating stories, and arguing with loved ones.
- Turn down the lights. Ensure that your room is dark or use a sleep mask. Ideally, remove all devices from the bedroom. TVs, cell phones, or computers in the bedroom can be a distraction and deprive you of much-needed sleep. If that is not possible, then cease exposure to all screens as far in advance as possible

before bed, but ideally, one to two hours or more before lying down to initiate sleep.

- Keep your bedroom on the cooler side. Our body temperature naturally drops at nighttime. Keeping the room cool helps expedite that process, getting us to fall asleep quicker and stay asleep longer.
- Try expressive writing. Take five to ten minutes (longer if you like) to write down anything that comes to mind—thoughts, feelings, wishes, or any other ideas. Use paper or a journal rather than a device. Don't worry about spelling, grammar, or punctuation. Just write. Depending on preference, you can write and retain (keep in an ongoing journal) or divulge and dump (shred or throw out). Writing this way helps bring authentic emotion from your subconsciousness into your consciousness, lowering the autonomic nervous system stimulation required to inhibit these emotions (i.e., to keep them suppressed or repressed). Writing down feelings you may otherwise suppress will send strong messages of safety to your brain, allowing it to stop trying to "protect" you from letting these thoughts and feelings out) and help it relax (suppression of emotion sends messages of danger to the brain that those emotions are threatening and need to be concealed).
- Declutter your bedroom to get rid of anything that might distract from sleep, such as noises, lights, and uncomfortable sheets. To cope with unavoidable noises (snoring partners or sounds in your environment), consider wearing ear plugs.
- Face your clock away from you so you can't see the time. Often, and especially when we have trouble sleeping, seeing the time increases anxiety and impedes sleep.
- Avoid napping after 3 p.m. Naps can help sleep deficits, but late afternoon naps make it harder to fall asleep at night.
- Avoid caffeine and nicotine (both are stimulants). Coffee, sodas, teas, and chocolate are all culprits in causing insomnia. Nicotine causes smokers to sleep too lightly and wake up too early because of nicotine withdrawal.

- Avoid alcohol before bed, as it impairs REM sleep and keeps you in the lighter stages of sleep. If you are using alcohol to help you relax before bed, consider that you likely may wake up in the middle of the night when the alcohol wears off.
- Sleep-enhancing medication has been associated with increased mortality.[8] If you choose to go this route, discuss it with your physician and use it as a last resort for as short a period as possible.
- Avoid medicine (prescription and over-the-counter) that delays or disrupts sleep. Check with your pharmacist to see if you are taking anything that could be impacting your sleep. If that is the case, work with your doctor to adjust the medication or the time of ingestion to better support a good night's rest.

What about children and sleep? It is particularly challenging to support kids in a connected way when you are tired and under-resourced. Being prepared with some steps and options beforehand can make or break your connection, leaving you both either feeling wonderful or awful depending on how the situation is navigated.

We have found that when kids have a hard time falling asleep, there are two common issues.

1) They are scared of nightmares or other frightening thoughts. At WeHeal, we teach parents to help their children "transform" scary dreams and thoughts in such a way that the fear they otherwise induce is replaced with compassion and understanding. This results in the child experiencing a sense of safety, connection, and peace that will then support sleep.

2) They are dysregulated and need help calming their nervous system. Contrary to popular parenting practices, firmly demanding that your child calm down and go to sleep does anything but help them feel calm. We know this from our own experience because that used to be our only tool, and despite its ineffectiveness, we continued hoping that each time we used it, it would deliver a

different result. Our growing frustration led us to develop a wonderful tool we call the "body calmer." We start by taking thirty seconds to close our eyes (both parent and child) and check into our body to see where we are on the "Check-In-Meter" (see diagram below or Appendix G). A "10" means we feel super hyper or jittery and can't sit still whereas a "1" means we feel really calm, open, and peaceful inside. We like to emphasize that there is no "right" number and what matters most is being honest with where you are. Often, we share our number out loud, although it works just as well if you keep it to yourself.

Once we have our number, we begin the Body Calmer exercise. The idea is to connect a movement you enjoy to your breath. Our favorite exercise is tracing each other's hands. To do this, begin by walking your finger up your thumb (or your child's) as you breathe in and then down the thumb as you breathe out SLOWLY. It helps to hear the breath out as it makes it easier to ensure that it is happening slowly. This is repeated on each finger on the front of one hand, then the back of one hand, and then again on the other hand, front and then back. If you went first as the parent tracing the child's fingers, have them switch and trace each of your fingers. Breathe in together as they trace up your first finger, then breathe out together, SLOWLY, as they trace down that finger. Repeat this again on all fingers on the one hand, front and back, and then switch to the other hand, front and back. Once both of you have completed this, together you will have taken forty breaths in, with forty slow exhales out. Now it is time to use the Check-In-Meter again to gauge where we are. Again, there is no right number (it could have even gone up), as the goal is to just check in to your body and use a number to define where you are. That's it. We find that one of our children loves doing this regularly, whereas the other prefers to do this only when feeling really revved up. The key is to make it work for them and be something enjoyable—connecting and regulating that can be done together. Helping your child regulate is important in delivering messages of safety and feeling safe is vital to a good night's sleep.

Check-in Meter

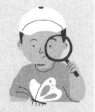

10 My mind and body are jumping all around.

9

8 My mind is busy and my body is tense.

7

6 My mind is moving and my body is uncomfortable.

5

 My mind is cloudy and my body is softening.

4

3 My mind is clearing and my body is calming.

2

1 My mind and body are calm, peaceful, and open.

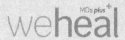

At WeHeal, we offer additional opportunities to improve sleep hygiene using our EoW model. For more detailed information, please refer to the individual chapters designated for these topics.

1) Self: Remember that through suppression and repression, we convey to ourselves that who we are (our full authentic self) is dangerous. Taking time to connect with our authentic self is a profound way of decreasing threat and signifying to the body that we are safe. It is not enough to cognitively understand that we are safe; to truly exit survival mode, we need to signal to our body, through actions and not thoughts, that we are safe.
   - Practice self-empathy and compassion
   - Engage in self-regulating techniques such as cognitive soothing and somatic tracking, meditation, breath exercises, music, and dance or yoga
   - Try expressive writing

2) Nutrition: Pursue a healthy body weight by choosing calorie-dilute, nutrient dense foods.
   - Extra weight can make breathing comfortably more challenging while sleeping. And obesity is an identified risk factor for sleep apnea.
   - Avoid large meals at night. Meals that leave us feeling stuffed and are too close to bedtime can cause reflux, which can impede sleep.
   - Limit, or eliminate, processed and fatty foods at dinnertime, as they can increase reflux and bloating.
   - If hunger is preventing you from sleeping, consider a healthy light snack like fruit.
   - If you make frequent night-time trips to the bathroom, consider curbing your fluid intake in the late afternoon and evening. Nighttime awakenings result in fragmented and impaired sleep.

3) Activity: Daily physical activity is essential for optimal sleep health and is associated with better sleep. Aim for thirty minutes per day, ideally no later than two to three hours before bed.
   - Avoid vigorous evening exercise, as that can stimulate the nervous system, making it harder to fall asleep.
   - Weather permitting, go outside. Outdoor light exposure supports the health of your natural circadian rhythm (the internal process that regulates the sleep-wake cycle and repeats roughly every twenty-four hours). Daylight is key to regulating sleep patterns, so try to get outside for at least thirty minutes each day (or one hour, if you struggle to fall asleep).

4) Play: Ensure daily participation in activities that are purposeless, all-consuming, and fun, without the need to accomplish any required goals. Free play sends powerful safety messages to the brain, especially the subconscious, which is constantly running predictive codes and algorithms to assess if you are safe or in danger. The safer we feel, the better we sleep.
   - Find your favorite ways to play and make space for them daily. Even five to ten minutes a day can make a profound impact. If you don't have time to spare, then incorporate play in your daily activities. Try singing as you wash the dishes or while on the drive home, dancing with the housework or out the door to work, or racing the kids to see who can fold the laundry the fastest.

5) Connection: Optimizing connection with your external world is one of the most significant ways to meet needs for safety and security. And safety-enhancing (threat-reducing) activities are an essential part of sleep hygiene.
   - When disconnected from your most important relationships (even if subconsciously), your brain perceives a threat, and over time, this becomes the norm. If the brain is in threat mode during the day, it is hard to shut that off when you want

to sleep. Safety messages during the day allow the brain to feel safe and welcome sleep at night.

- Contributing to society and our greater world is an important need of every person, but it is often overlooked when we are stuck in the day-to-day survival state. Your brain will not focus on meaning, purpose, and contribution to others when it feels it is under threat. By intentionally pursuing meaning, purpose, and contribution, you send messages of safety that your brain can receive. Remember, your brain assesses safety by experience, not by what you tell it.

> "Sleep is an investment in the energy
> you need to be effective tomorrow."
>
> —Tom Roth

Sleep is the single most effective way to wipe your health slate clean each day. When you rest and restore your body, you set your day in motion to ensure Life Is Wonderful.

CHAPTER 12

Connection: The Missing Key to Optimal Health

"We human beings are social beings. We come into
the world as the result of others' actions. We survive
here in dependence on others. Whether we like it or
not, there is hardly a moment of our lives when we do
not benefit from others' activities. For this reason, it is
hardly surprising that most of our happiness arises in
the context of our relationships with others."

—DALAI LAMA

HUMAN CONNECTION PLAYS a crucial role in our health and well-being. Disconnection and the resulting isolation we experience are among the main triggers of danger signals in our body. As discussed in the chapter that introduced polyvagal theory (Chapter 6), when our body perceives threat, it triggers a cascade of physiological changes that include shifts in our autonomic nervous system towards a state of reactivity and fighting/fleeing, an extensive proinflammatory cytokine release, and release of a host of chemicals including adrenaline, cortisol, and histamine.

In a 1988 report, James House and colleagues summarized multiple studies starting in the '60s and '70s in the United States, Finland, and Sweden, in total accounting for more than 40,000 people followed up over a period ranging from 5 to 13 years, looking at the effects social isolation has on health and mortality. These studies showed that, after controlling for other variables, lack of connection (having social relationship(s) involving close contact where you can authentically share your most private feelings and needs) increased a person's risk of illness. In fact, people in good health who were disconnected were twice as likely to die as people of similar health who experienced connection with others.[1]

If connection is crucial for our health and well-being, then getting more clarity around the concept seems worthwhile. Connection is a certain quality of felt experience between two or more people. It happens when we offer ourselves to each other free of judgments. It's when the innocence behind any regrettable words or actions is warmly acknowledged, and our limitations are tenderly understood. In this space, we experience being seen and heard on a heart level. And being heard this way contributes to the felt sense that our experience is valid, that it counts, and that we matter. When our experience is validated in this way, so is our very existence. That leaves us feeling safe and provides a sense of inner peace and comfort. Connection is how we become a source of healing, nourishment, and strength for each other. And it's why being in this state has an unmistakable quality of harmony and flow.

There are times when connection with others comes easy. But in times of conflict, or when triggered, connection can be very challenging. Let's face it, relationships can get messy! That's especially the case when we don't see eye to eye. When we're deeply triggered by something someone has done, trying to see that person's innocence or good intentions feels like the last thing we want to do, right? And simply trying to use a "nice" voice to resolve a conflict is a poor substitute for being in connection. When we are in connection, something magical happens; hearts are opened and heard and there's a felt sense of harmony with the other. Remarkably enough, when we enjoy harmony and resonance, we can still have peace and warmth despite having unresolved issues with that person.

We obviously want to resolve our conflicts. But when we put conflict resolution before connection, we run the risk of having the conversation feel similar to business negotiations from across the table. At that point, the best we can achieve is compromise, which is a nice way of saying everyone loses a little. Even when we find solutions this way, what remains is disconnection, a sentiment of separation and scarcity. However, when we establish connection first, we find ourselves on the same side of the table, with a genuine interest in finding mutual solutions that work both ways. It becomes a "together project," similar to working on an old-fashioned board puzzle with someone—sharing and comparing pieces to find a fit that works.

Prioritizing connection with dishes after dinner

When the quality of connection is prioritized before strategizing, then natural shifting can occur between two people so that both parties win. In Nonviolent Communication (NVC), we tell people to not do something unless you can do it with the joy a child feels when feeding a hungry duck. We use something called the "duck meter" (created by CNVC Certified Trainer, Ike Lasater), in which ten ducks means that you experience a lot of joy in doing something and less than seven ducks means you experience little to no joy. The numbers seven, eight, and nine hold a unique position of conveying a continuum of willingness to joyful.

In our family, we don't want people to agree to do anything if there are less than seven ducks on the duck meter. Our desire is to give willingly and not out of obligation or perceived duty, because anything we do out of obligation gets stored in a "you owe me" box. As we continue to show up obligingly, that box gets more and more stuffed, until it explodes in the form of reactivity, anger, disconnection, or even violence.

Many parents might worry that this strategy is permissive. If we don't make our children do things, they won't want to do anything. With NVC, however, there is a trust that shifting can occur when we connect around our underlying needs and care for one another. As parents, we inherently care about our children and have compassion for them. Similarly, children naturally care about their parents and want to support them as well.

Our story: Dishes after dinner

When we finish dinner, we ask our children if they would be willing to help clear the table. Our request is to not say yes unless there are seven or more ducks. Hearing and trusting that they have choice represents the first step in creating a quality of connection in which shifting can happen. Kylee and Jordan often test this out by saying they are at a five; we respond with "Don't do any more unless it's at least a seven. However, before you decide, would you be willing to hear how clearing the dishes contributes to us?" They are almost always willing to hear, at which point we share that their contribution helps preserve our energy for other things like playing after dinner. Or we might share that we are feeling really tired and the contribution would support our needs for ease and help. Again, almost always, after they hear how their actions would contribute to making our lives more wonderful, they are more than willing to shift to a seven or more. The key here is that their shift resulted from choice and their actions were contributed willingly. In order for this to work, it is imperative that all parties trust that 1) there is a natural desire for us, as humans, to contribute to each other, and if we don't do so, there is generally a really good reason; and, 2) there will not be consequences or punishments for times where there is unwillingness to shift.

If connection is a skill that can be learned and improved with practice, where do we start? To answer this question, we can look to the work of Marshall Rosenberg, the founder of the Center for Nonviolent Communication. In his book *Nonviolent Communication,*[2] Rosenberg offers a framework and way of relating that brings a considerable degree of clarity, precision, and order to the skill of connecting. This chapter presents a broad, conceptual overview on connection based on Rosenberg's framework and his key principles. And the chapters that follow will focus on applying the framework and key principles within the context of family life, friends, work, spirituality, and our natural world.

Rosenberg wasn't alone in seeing human needs as the driving force behind human behavior. Albert Einstein, in an article entitled *Religion and Science* in the New York Times, shared a similar understanding:

> *"Everything that the human race has done and thought is concerned with the satisfaction of deeply felt needs and the assuagement of pain. One has to keep this constantly in mind if one wishes to understand spiritual movements and their development. Feeling and longing are the motive force behind all human endeavor and human creation, in however exalted a guise the latter may present themselves to us."*[3]

What are needs?

According to the Center for Nonviolent Communication, "The word *needs* refers to *Universal Human Needs*, which are defined as: the conditions necessary for life to thrive in any human being, regardless of culture or geography; core human motivators which impel us to act; how Life is seeking to show up in this moment—in you or me or any person; energies that want to flow, not holes to be filled."[4]

On the other hand, strategies are defined as the ways we go about meeting needs. They are not universal and may vary from person to person. So, while we all share the same needs, we may take very different actions to meet those needs. Understanding this difference is essential, because only strategies come into conflict, not needs. When we focus on needs, we can identify many different strategies to meet those needs arising in that moment between people.

Regardless of our culture, ethnicity, race, or gender, human beings share the same basic needs, wants, longings, desires, and values. Consider the list below. It is by no means exhaustive.

NEEDS	
Acceptance/Belonging	Kindness
Affection/Care	Mourning
Appreciation	Movement
Autonomy/Choice	Mutuality
Celebration	Nourishment
Clarity	Nurturing
Comfort	Order
Compassion	Partnership
Competence	Peace
Consideration	Play
Contribution	Reassurance
Ease	Respect
Fairness	Rest
Friendship	Safety
Health	Security
Honesty	Support
Hope	To be Heard
Independence	To Matter
Integrity	Trust
Joy	Understanding

At different times and to varying degrees, the above qualities are the driving force behind all our actions. Don't take our word for it. Carefully consider what moves you to speak and act throughout your day. This will require that we slow down and bring a measure of mindful awareness to our daily activities and interactions with others.

Begin to take notice of what it is you want when you approach your loved ones in conversation. Are you wanting to contribute to their well-being with warmth and care? Or are you craving a little affection and attention from them at that moment? What pulls you to turn on a movie or a TV show? Are you wanting engagement, inspiration or, maybe, escape? What draws you to the refrigerator? Is it sheer hunger, or wanting to meet needs for health and sustenance? Or are you feeling restless or bored and are you edging to the fridge for stimulation, comfort, or release? If you practice slowing down and becoming aware of what needs lie behind your words and actions, moment by moment, you open up to a new world of self-discovery, self-understanding, and clarity. And, as will become clear, knowing what we need or value in a given situation is an integral part of improving our ability to connect to others and to ourselves.

When we understand more about our feelings, emotions, desires, and motivations, we improve our connection skills. We have an instinctive tendency to look outside ourselves, in response to how we feel, to identify the culprit or perpetrator. Did they make us angry, sad, frustrated, or scared? Did they betray, misunderstand, or hurt us? This seems perfectly understandable, given how our species evolved. Those who survived placed immediate attention on the external circumstances that triggered their internal experiences (i.e., feelings, emotions, sensations) and instinctive responses. Life-saving reactions, not armchair reflections, preserved our predecessors on the African plains. In survival mode, there is no time to discern if we need safety or reassurance; when we see the tiger, we run! And yet, as we continue to evolve from merely surviving to thriving within our more modern civilization, we have the luxury to delve into our emotional experiences and to become more aware of how and why they come to be. Through mindful awareness, we have the ability to witness that it's our needs and values and the way we interpret events—the story we tell ourselves— that give rise to what we feel and how we experience life.

Consider the following example: Imagine you're driving and the car in the lane next to you suddenly cuts you off. You barely avoid an accident by slamming on your brakes and swerving out of the way. After the initial shock, you naturally feel frustration and anger, possibly even rage, as you tell yourself what a careless, thoughtless lunatic that driver is. Pause the story: It's important to note that the experience of frustration and anger actually comes from the story that the driver is a careless lunatic and from your needs for consideration and safety. Now imagine that, after being cut off, you look closely into that car and see that the driver is actually slumped over and two small children are in the backseat, crying hysterically. Pause the story again: Notice now how your emotional landscape quickly changes in combination with your needs for compassion, support, and care. The new story becomes that you are dealing with an out-of-control car and the family is in trouble; the driver may have suffered a heart attack. Your new experience is one of great concern for their welfare, not one of frustration and anger.

Now, from the comfort of your reading chair, notice what happens within you if you imagine that the driver lost consciousness *only after* "intentionally" cutting you off. Of course, you'd still care about their safety. But, do you also notice a subtle shift back to irritation and indignation toward the driver? That is because our feelings about the driver and of the situation are relative to what story we tell ourselves, our perception and how that affects our own needs and values. Which brings us to the point: our felt experience of a given circumstance, our perception, is ultimately based upon internal factors, not external ones. And those feelings can change by the second as the story or narrative changes along with the needs that are arising in that moment. This is an objective fact about our subjective, emotional experience. And it's this objective fact that allows us to take responsibility for ALL of our feelings that arise in response to OUR needs from OUR "chosen" (often subconscious) narrative or story we tell ourselves in the moment.

Can we honestly say that others can't make us feel anything? Let's take a harder example then. Bring to your mind someone with whom spending time is challenging. Got a person? Okay, now imagine that he/she does that "thing" you don't like, right in front of you. You've already had conversations with this person about this thing and how you dislike it. What is more, leading up to that moment, this individual has been acting differently toward you and barely speaking. And, when this person does the thing you dislike, he/she makes direct eye contact with you. Getting the emotional flavor here? Tasting notes of frustration with not-so-subtle hints of resentment?

It's absolutely true that knowing the cultural customs and social etiquette in a given context and having a basic understanding of human nature, we can have a pretty good idea what might trigger a person. And it almost goes without saying that those closest to us know best how to get on our nerves! Nonetheless, in the above example, isn't it equally true to say that the frustration and resentment were a direct result of *our* interpretation of that person's actions and how those actions affected *our* needs for care, consideration, and understanding? And wouldn't it be more accurate to say those were *our* emotions, not the other person's, based upon *our* values and needs in that moment, not theirs? If we didn't have those needs, that story, or both, we wouldn't have that experience.

This dynamic is best exemplified when we consider a stimulus that can generate two different feelings, depending on the situation. For example, let's say you were expecting someone for a meeting and they were fifteen minutes late. If you are making last minute preps for the meeting, you might be grateful for the fifteen-minute grace period. On the other hand, if you have another meeting scheduled right after, you might be annoyed at the fifteen-minute delay. If the stimulus, in this case fifteen minutes, was the cause of your emotions, you would consistently feel the same way about it. However, the reality is that our response is a result of needs that come up for us regardless of the stimulus. My needs in the moment, not the other person's actions, are what cause my feelings. Looking at the first scenario, enjoying more time to prepare for the meeting, your needs may have been time, space, competence, completion, and ease. In contrast, in the second scenario where you got upset, your needs may have been reliability, integrity, and consideration. As we'll see, owning this process allows us to maintain internal integrity and take a better approach.

So why is it important to take responsibility for our own emotions, especially when every bone in our body wants to blame and shame the trigger? We have two main reasons. First, when we attribute the cause of our feelings to external factors, we effectively give away our power and our peace of mind. This externalization of our emotional experience is what we do when we blame. Second, we have another, better option when triggered. We can look inside as we process our emotionally charged experience, focus our attention on what it is we want or value in that moment, and address the situation from that energetic state.

This move inward typically increases our sense of choice, increasing our likelihood that we'll respond to what it is we want, rather than react to what we don't want. For example, if we perceive that our partner is speaking to us without respect, we could choose to blame and shame them for hurting us by being rude and disrespectful. But we have a choice. Instead of focusing on all the actions that we don't want to experience, we can take inventory on what it is that we *do* want: respect, kindness, and consideration.

Focusing on our own needs, when triggered, reminds us that *we* are responsible for them, not another person. And taking responsibility in this way is liberating because there is more than one way for us to meet the same need. For example, some people meet their need for safety by living with friends; others meet that same need by installing an alarm system; and still others do so by owning a gun. When we realize there are many ways to meet our needs, our world becomes infinitely more expansive. For these reasons, when we own our needs as well as acknowledge the many different ways to meet our needs, we're able to retain a sense of agency, power, and a form of emotional integrity. Going external and blaming a person or situation operates on an implicit and often unconscious belief that we can't feel better until those external conditions are changed. Unfortunately, this dynamic brings with it the tragic strategy of trying to control the behavior of others. For example, we want to make them stop being "rude" or "disrespectful." Believing that what we feel is a result of external factors fosters a sense of helplessness since we can't always change those factors or make others do what we want, without compromising connection. Alternatively, we can shift from trying to force and coerce other people to meet our needs to finding our internal power to meet our own needs in other ways.

The next time you get triggered and find yourself blaming the situation or the other person involved, bring in some mindful awareness. Don't try to change your experience or criticize yourself for blaming—just observe. See if you notice feelings of despair and helplessness along with your other emotions. Notice if you find yourself wanting to react in order to regain power. Many people feel that they can't stand the experience of helplessness or despair, so they try to regain a sense of power through anger or rage. When our needs are not being met or we worry they won't be met in the future, then it is easy to experience that perception as a threat, quickly followed by anger in an effort to control the unwanted outcome. Given our evolutionary heritage, the anger move is understandable. Anger signals danger and mobilizes our fight-or-flight survival instincts. The problem with anger, however, is that it typically comes at a very high cost to the relationship, and it doesn't foster connection. Anger is useful in that it tells us that an important need is not being satisfied. At the same time, though, responding with anger implies judging someone as the culprit or perpetrator; it gives away our power. Focusing instead on what it is we want or value when triggered is the practice of self-connection that allows us to maintain our integrity and agency. This is accomplished by connecting to the needs we hope to satisfy with the abundance of strategies available to us. Doing so will take time and practice but is vital in our quest for connection and a better outcome.

Taking responsibility is the most effective way to be authentic about our experience and express it in a way that still maintains connection. When triggered, we desperately want to be understood. But the means that we go about getting that understanding can sometimes be tragically counterproductive. Some of us may begin talking very loudly, as if the louder we get, the more likely the other person will be to "hear" and understand us. Other times we may attempt to get understanding for our pain by trying to create pain for the other person. In a roundabout way, having the other person experience some degree of pain is a way to get confirmation that our own pain is felt, acknowledged, appreciated, and shared. Or we may resort to blame, accusations, and judgments in a roundabout way of expressing our unmet needs. And then other times, ironically, we will not talk at all to try to be heard, which is also known as shutting down. We have all resorted to these strategies at one point or another in our lives and, to some degree, still resort to these ways to be heard and healed. Unfortunately, they are as tragically ineffective at meeting most of our needs as they are detrimental to fostering connection.

When we can acknowledge that what we're feeling is based on what we're telling ourselves about the situation and what it is we value and want, we keep the ball in our own court and people are more willing to engage with us. In other words, when we take responsibility for our own feelings and needs and make our emotional experience about us, people usually respond in a less defensive way, resulting in a greater willingness to truly hear us and contribute to our needs. Which would you respond to better: "you are so rude and inconsiderate, don't talk to me like that!" or "I am needing more respect and consideration, would you be willing to say that differently?" The latter version increases not only the likelihood that we will stay in connection but also the possibility that our needs will be met. Although this practice takes time to integrate, the rewards can be felt immediately. Connecting in this way not only feels better to the other person—it feels better to us.

Let's consider those sentences again: "you are so rude and inconsiderate, don't talk to me like that!" Notice how your body, and possibly that of the person you are speaking to, feels a little tighter and more mobilized. Then imagine saying, "I am needing more respect and consideration, would you be willing to say that differently?" Communicating this way, you may notice some subtle softening in both yourself and the person you are speaking with. That difference you see and feel may be subtle at first but with growing self-connection and self-awareness, you will experience an even greater contrast, and impact, between connecting and disconnecting language.

Matt's Story

Early on in my training I asked my Nonviolent Communication assessor, Sylvia Haskvitz, why I needed to talk to a customer service agent with kindness and respect if they keep making mistakes and transferring me to different agents. After all, when that happens, I feel upset and want to express my anger. Plus, I won't talk to them again, so what need of mine does that really meet? She responded by asking me to notice how I feel in my body when I talk to an agent in a way that is congruent with my value of kindness and respect compared to talking to an agent in ways that are not in integrity with those same values. It was clear as day: my body was tighter, and underneath the anger that was fueling responses that lacked kindness and respect, there was sadness and disappointment. In other words, connecting language is as much for me as it is for the person with whom I am connecting. As you become more self-connected, this will be ever more apparent and empowering. That awareness of how it feels in my body is so much more reinforcing than being nice simply because that is the "right" way to treat people.

We've all had the experience of being in conflict with someone and thinking to ourselves, "How can he see it that way? That's so off-base!" All the same, another key component to keeping connection open is respecting everyone's perspective (i.e., the stories we have). To tell someone that his/her perspective is inaccurate, foolish, unreasonable, or anything along those lines will, for most of us, kill connection right on the spot. The fact is, there are times we realize that what we're telling ourselves is neither reasonable nor true! Even when we realize this, if the individual with whom we're in conflict were to discount our story as "unreasonable," we may no longer feel safe to connect. So long as a story triggers pain in us or another, we must hold it with respect, regardless of its substance. This is the most constructive thing we can do to keep connection open. It is not the truth of their story that matters; rather, it is the pain in their heart as a result of their story or perception that matters. Whether you believe the story is true or not, accurate or inaccurate, their pain is real and in need of care. Connection means caring more about what is in someone's heart than what is coming out of their mouth.

While respecting each person's perspective keeps connection open, it's moving toward what we have in common that connects us. We all share the same fundamental needs. And as just explained, emotional experience—whether pleasant or unpleasant—is the result of the story we tell ourselves and whether, in that moment, we experience our needs to be met or unmet. So, when we respectfully hold a person's perspective and understand from within that perspective how needs aren't being met, we have the means to lean into that person's pain with compassion. We may not agree with that person's take on the situation. In fact, we may find that person's point of view triggering! But differentiating ourselves from the other person's needs allows us to connect to how understandable it would be for that person to have certain feelings based on his/her perspective on the matter.

What's remarkable here is how we can still have meaningful connection even when our points of view are different. This requires that we learn how to hold another's point of view, no matter how much we disagree with it, without getting hung up on it. The more we can make our children's or partner's anger about their needs instead of something we did wrong, the easier it will be to connect. This approach allows us to focus on what is going on inside of them, instead of explaining ourselves (and getting defensive) or pointing out why they were to blame and not us (shifting blame).

Just as critical as not getting hung up over perspectives is not getting hung up in moralistic judgment over words or actions that we don't like. We lose connection to our shared humanity when we judge words or actions against standards such as right or wrong, good or bad, appropriate or inappropriate. We lose sight of the innocence behind the intention of an action, yet that is essential to make compassion possible. To stay in connection, we need compassion. And to have compassion, we need to stay grounded in our shared humanity by connecting with the human needs and/or values that motivate a person's words or deeds.

Now at times, we may strongly dislike the choices that others make. We may even take a strong stance against certain behaviors. In other words, it is not that we should not ever judge; rather, we may use judgment to discern what meets our own needs versus what doesn't. The reason to avoid speaking in absolute moralistic judgment terms is because it disconnects us from others. For example, it may not meet your needs for safety and kindness to hit another person. Sharing that truth is much more connecting than simply saying hitting is wrong. It is important to share your values, with the most effective and uniting way to do so being to connect with the other person around their impact on YOU versus judging them, blaming them, labeling them as wrong, or stimulating shame. Ultimately, when we stay connected to the needs or values, we still have access to compassion for others and therefore the possibility of connection remains open. It is essential that people understand that communicating this way or thinking this way is not the "right way" or "better way"; rather, it is what we have found to be the most likely to lead to connection. And when we are more connected, there is a greater chance of being in the state of perceived safety, which includes a physiological, chemical, and neurological shift in your body towards growth, restoration, and healing. So, it not only feels better emotionally and spiritually but it feels better physically and is what allows you to live in the state of Life Is Wonderful.

On the other hand, compassion goes offline when we lose sight of our shared humanity and judge people based on right and wrong. This is accompanied by a physiological shift in our body towards danger and threat. When we relate to others based upon such standards and we determine that a person has fallen short, to some degree, we turn against that person. We become more geared toward protection and punishment. Remember the example of the driver who cut us off. When we imagined being intentionally cut off, our feelings turned against that driver. To the degree that we find ourselves stuck in judgments toward others, we'll no longer want connection with them. When we impede connection, we not only stimulate pain in others, we hurt ourselves. We'll find ourselves wanting to blame, shame, or do worse. So the question remains, when we find ourselves stuck in judgment, how do we get our compassion back?

Let's be honest, when we're stuck in judgments and/or flooded with challenging emotions, we're typically not asking ourselves how we can regain compassion and enter back into connection. The habitual tendency is to externalize and blame, which is often done at least in part to protect us from a sense of vulnerability and pain. In other words, it is our subconscious mind's well-intentioned way of trying to protect us. So, the first step in the direction of compassion is to turn toward our inner experience with kindness and understanding, bringing a soft and warm acceptance to our charged and uncomfortable, emotional experience as well as the pain of our unmet needs, and reminding ourselves that judgments are natural, not negative.

It can also be helpful to regain some perspective by making it clear to ourselves that our judgment isn't reality. One practical way of separating ourselves from our judgments (giving ourselves a little room to respond differently) is to restate the judgmental thought from something like, "He's so selfish!" to "*I am telling myself* that he's so selfish." Restating our judgments in terms of something we're telling ourselves typically brings more openness and objectivity around the judgmental message. This allows us to create some distance from our judgment while forming a healthy measure of doubt around its reality.

Once we've brought a measure of warmth and acceptance to our inner experience, we can use our judgment to learn more about ourselves. Though it may not be initially apparent because of their outwardly focused and negatively charged nature, judgments can tell us what we value or need. So, the next step toward regaining our compassion is to remove the judgment's protective armor and find the precious need or value that's beneath. For example, let's say I have the following judgment: "*This person doesn't give a damn about me!*" Behind this, I could have quite a few needs. But for simplicity's sake, let's just say my most tender needs here are for *care* and *consideration*. Essentially, I want the sense that people care about me and that I matter in the equation. This is the vulnerable reality behind the armor.

Knowing the vulnerable truth behind my judgment, I can connect to what is precious in me: my needs for care and consideration. You might ask, "How will connecting to what is precious bring back compassion?"

The fact is, moving beneath the hard, protective exterior into the undefended, warmth of our universal needs uncovers our own innocence. We find a "child" that is sad or scared and that's hiding, not knowing if it matters to other people and wondering how to ask for what it wants. Spending even a few seconds focusing on this beauty can have a pronounced softening effect on our felt experience. Once we've touched our own humanity in this way, we may have the reserves to turn our attention to the other person's humanity. And looking beyond our moralistic judgment as to what is precious and vulnerable in the other person's actions or words brings our compassion back online, which rekindles our desire to connect. This could look like making a guess as to what is going on inside the other person when they made the comment that stimulated you to think, "they don't give a damn about me." What needs do you imagine they were trying to meet with their actions? Does naming their needs give you a better understanding, and maybe even some compassion, for their chosen strategy to meet those needs?

At this point, it's worth noting that, even after connecting with our own or another's beauty and innocence, it isn't uncommon for a moralistic judgment about the other person to re-emerge with vigor. It's almost as if the judgment pushes its way back to the forefront of our consciousness, waving its hands, jumping up and down, pointing fingers, and blaming all over again. That is simply old habitual processes popping back up to protect us from pain and helping us get our needs met. However, trying to connect with that person's innocence while still feeling judgmental may seem incongruent or unnatural.

Understanding authenticity allows us to meet our need for congruency even when we find our internal, emotional state a challenge. Being authentic doesn't mean giving unfiltered expressions of our judgmental thoughts, as that runs counter to our primary objective to focus on connection above all else. It means responding in a way that meets the majority of our own needs and values, while caring about the needs of others.

When we react based on our judgmental thoughts, it leaves many of our needs unmet (peace of mind, compassion, care, warmth, contribution, effectiveness, growth, integrity, love, respect, kindness). And yet the habitual tendency and energetic charge of a judgment makes our quest for authenticity far from smooth sailing. For this reason, being true to ourselves may require a higher degree of intentionality, determination, and skill. And knowing what it means to be truly authentic may help to steady our hand and fortify our conviction to meet as many of our needs and values as possible in the heat of the moment, instead of meeting some of our needs at the expense of others.

Furthermore, depending on how stuck we feel, we may need support from another. In an almost magical way, being viewed with compassion and understanding by another increases our own ability to see ourselves in that same warm light. Therefore, we may first need to receive empathy and compassion from someone else to reconnect to our own innocence and power. Ultimately, though, the path back to compassion for, and connection with, the person we're judging remains the same and involves us seeing that person's beauty and innocence (the very needs they were trying to meet with their actions).

As previously stated, when we slow down and carefully observe what drives our own words and deeds, we realize that everything we do (or don't do) is an attempt to meet universal needs, longings, and values. Simply put, we are always trying to meet our needs with everything we say, think, or do. Whether it's working a job, listening to music, going to church, browsing on social media, avoiding a coworker, having dessert, meditating, giving to charity, or anything else, it all can be traced back to the same beautiful source: trying to meet needs. We gain a valuable shift in perspective when we begin to understand that we are all doing the best we can with the capacity, skill, and awareness we have at that moment. We may not have concrete proof of this, but we do know that Life Is Wonderful when we see the world through this lens!

In reality, we don't choose what we need at a given moment. Needs, longings, and desires simply arise from within us, moment by moment, typically in response to our conditioning and the particular context in which we find ourselves. Practices such as mindfulness and meditation can help make this realization more concrete and the awareness of our needs easier to discern and sort. And while our needs may be somewhat predictable within the scope of our daily routines, we can't make ourselves feel (or not feel) something, let alone need or value something. While our needs and values are always present, when and to what degree they give us their energetic momentum is ultimately something that is witnessed, not willed.

When we are willing to do something, it resonates with our life's energy and the needs that arise at that time. And if we're not willing, it means we have another need that has a stronger energetic momentum. Our willingness can change in a second, however, in light of a new idea, a memory or thought, a request from another, or a different set of circumstances. And while it's true that we can generally predict what may potentially move us or others to action, energetic shifts are not a given. The same set of circumstances that affected our willingness one day may not have the same effect the next, even if we wished it did. The implications here are both profound and practical in relation to connection.

Given that we don't control our needs or values, we could say they're ultimately expressions and movements of the energy of life working through us—of the force that keeps all things going. So, when I have a need or longing for something, understanding and accepting that need becomes essential to understanding and accepting life as it is. Our focus then is to better understand the energy that moves us and to work with, not against, it. When we can acknowledge and work with this energy in others, and not get sideswiped by how it's sometimes expressed or lived, we stay in connection and experience the beautiful flow of this energy of life. And thus we come full circle: to stay in connection is to stay in harmony and resonance, not just with ourselves and others, but with life itself.

Positive gossip

A fun connection exercise is called positive gossiping. You ask one person to turn their back to you as you proceed to talk with the group about them behind their back. However, you are talking about all the ways they meet your needs, all of the pleasant feelings they stimulate, and all of the gratitude and celebration you have around them. You continue to take turns sharing about them, talking as if they aren't even there.

Matt's perspective

For example, if Alona's back was to the group, I might say, "One thing I really like about Alona is how hard she works and her dedication to writing this book. It really gives me a sense of trust and peace knowing that she is in charge and going to get this project to the finish line. I feel so happy and appreciative of her efforts and contribution." Then someone else might say, "Yeah, that Alona, she is just so kind and caring as she always tries her best to share feedback with me with a gentle tone and warmth, even if it is about something she doesn't enjoy. I am so glad to be working on her team." And so on and so forth. It is fun to record this so the person being gossiped about can listen to it again in the future. Since many people have a hard time taking in wholehearted appreciation when looking you in the eyes, this is a wonderful and fun way to share it in a way that can more easily be received. Give it a try on your family or work team and see how much fun it is to build connection this way.

CHAPTER 13

Family and Friends

Pillar 6

"The strongest love is the love
that can demonstrate its fragility."
—PAULO COELHO

LIVING IN CONNECTION BEGINS with vulnerability. Vulnerability means showing your underbelly, exposing what is inside of you, what is alive in your heart. In essence, it shows your truth without editing, polishing, or airbrushing it in an effort to make it more socially acceptable and harmonious. What's more, this "essence" inside of you is magnetic, attracting other people's essence in a way that creates a deep and meaningful quality of connection. It is from within this "quality of connection" that healing, collaboration, and compassionate giving and receiving occur naturally. In a culture where "having it all together" is prized, being vulnerable about our ups and downs in life can be both unnerving and daunting. And yet, when it comes to connecting to others, being vulnerable about what we're feeling or needing actually demonstrates a real strength and power. How can this be? Knowing what we feel, value, or need at a given moment requires a significant level of self-awareness, self-care, self-respect, and, to some extent, even self-acceptance. Those are emotional muscles not everyone has, especially when faced with challenging or uncomfortable emotions.

Ironically, even though our culture's subliminal message is that pleasant emotions are good, while unpleasant or challenging ones are bad, many are drawn to those who share their challenging experiences or emotions vulnerably. It touches that part of us that we all have in common but are often too afraid to share. Because of the pervasive cultural message, many simply don't know how to meet their need for acceptance, emotional safety, and authenticity. The leap is just too great. To those who would like to be more authentic in their close personal relationships, consider this idea: start where you are and start small. Try sharing, with someone you trust, an experience or emotion that is mildly challenging for you. In the following example, Tom will attempt sharing more vulnerably with Paul.

- **Paul:** Hey, Tom, how's your day going?
- **Tom:** Honestly, Paul, at the moment, I'm feeling a little unease. I just had a talk with my eldest son that didn't go as well as I would have liked.
- **Paul:** Huh, what happened? Everything okay with Billy?
- **Tom:** Oh yeah, it's nothing serious. I just have some regrets about the way Billy and I have been getting along these days. He's getting older faster than I realize sometimes and he just seems annoyed when I try to talk about the stuff we used to enjoy together. I feel a little sad about that. Wish we could talk with more warmth the way we used to. I miss that.
- **Paul:** Yeah, I bet, Tom. I hear your sadness and your wish for a warmer connection with Billy. That makes a lot of sense.
- **Tom:** Exactly. Thanks for listening, bud. I appreciate being able to be honest about it. That feels good.
- **Paul:** I appreciate you letting me in this way. We don't normally talk on this level, so I'm grateful you shared. Anytime you need a listening ear, I'm here.

Notice how Tom didn't pick a topic that was too overwhelming for either one of them. It was a current issue that had a manageable emotional charge behind it. And there was a level of trust that Paul would listen with care. All those factors are important when beginning to practice more authentic sharing. Starting where you are and starting small is the first step. The second step is choosing someone you trust to listen with care. When people share their emotional discomfort, they rarely want advice or even sympathy, as that tends to shut down rather than support deeper expression. Most just need their experience to be heard and understood. Notice how Paul responded to Tom's vulnerable expression with empathy and resonance, rather than with advice or sympathy.

When sharing struggles feels too challenging, another practice option is to try connecting vulnerably by sharing celebrations: pleasant emotions along with the needs that *are* being met (instead of starting with unpleasant emotions around needs that *are not* being met). For example, you could say, "When you gave me a hug just now, I felt really warm and tender and appreciated your care." Letting someone know how touched you are when you experience meeting a certain need or value you hold dear is a vulnerable expression. What's more, when you connect to your heart in that way, your entire body softens into the connection with yourself as well as with the person with whom you are sharing. This stimulates a deep sense of safety that shifts your physiology and body chemistry, which not only feels wonderful but also is extremely health promoting.

The well-known Zen Master Thich Nhat Hanh once said, "You listen with only one purpose: to help him or her to empty their heart." If a person is sharing his or her heart, then what that person needs is to be heard and understood. To give someone advice when what that person needs is to be heard is like giving him or her a hammer if the request is for a ladder. The result of misreading the need is often confusion and disconnection. So, getting straight in our mind what a person needs when he or she engages us in conversation represents an important step in keeping connection alive. The next step, as the Zen Master beautifully puts it, is to help that person empty their heart.

What is the best way to aid a person in emptying his or her heart? By simply listening, using body language that communicates that we're accompanying them wherever they need to go in the moment, and using resonant language—language of the heart that communicates to the other person that we get their emotional experience. By acknowledging what that person might be going through using feeling language rich with metaphor, imagery, and body sensations, we attempt to resonate with that person's emotional experience. In resonance, we sense support, and we don't feel alone. We can also offer guesses into what that person might be feeling or needing, empathizing further with that person's experience. And even if our empathy guesses are "off," our mere attempt still helps that person explore inward to confirm whether our guesses match his or her experience. The pain of unpleasant emotion is intensified when endured alone, so the heart naturally softens into accompaniment when a space is made without a desire to fix, educate, sympathize, cheer up, or deliver any other non-empathic response. Being aware of all of this may determine whether another person shuts down or openly empties their heart.

It's important to note, and learn to trust, that the point of empathy and resonance isn't to make people feel better or to solve their problems. This can be hard to get at first. We all want people who come to us, wanting to be heard, to feel better after we listen to them. This is natural and understandable on our part. Nonetheless, having this intention can very often lead to disappointment on both ends since the person's pain may have roots much deeper than are apparent given the issue presented. And if we listen to someone with the intention of helping that person to feel better, we carry with us a subtle agenda, even if it's a noble one, that can prevent us from being truly present for that person. People can sense that we have an agenda. And no one sharing their heart wants to be ushered along in that conversation to a particular emotional end for the sake of the listener. Thus, the goal when offering empathy and resonance is to simply be present and allow that person the safety and the space to empty his or her heart. Offering empathy is qualitatively different than offering sympathy to someone, even if the intention in both cases is to support that person. When we offer sympathy, we take the attention off that person and his or her experience and we place the focus of attention on our experience. So, while it can communicate care and be endearing, it runs the risk of disconnecting.

The following example will be one where Jessica gives Sandy sympathy about her situation. Can you sense disconnection happening as a result?

- **Jessica:** Hey Sandy, how are you? You don't look so happy.
- **Sandy:** I'm not, Jessica. I just had a fight with my boss and I'm not sure if I'll have a job tomorrow.
- **Jessica:** Sandy! Oh my gosh! I'm so sorry. That sucks. I feel so bad about that.
- **Sandy:** I'm actually worried sick. That job was so hard to get, and I really love what I'm doing there.
- **Jessica:** Geez... I'm truly sorry to hear it. I'm feeling scared for you too. I really hope things work out and your boss gets over it.
- **Sandy:** Yeah, me too.

Notice how Jessica communicated her care to her worried friend but kept the attention on herself. Sandy was feeling really worried and it's unclear whether Jessica's move to talk about her own emotional response really met Sandy's need to be heard, understood, and accompanied in her difficult moment.

Consider the same situation, except this time Jessica gives empathy and resonance to Sandy:

- **Jessica:** Hey Sandy, how are you? You don't look so happy.
- **Sandy:** I'm not, Jessica. I just had a fight with my boss and I'm not sure if I'll have a job tomorrow.
- **Jessica:** Oh my gosh Sandy, I'm imagining you're crawling out of your skin right now!
- **Sandy:** I am! I am worried sick! I love my job and I worked so hard to get it! I don't think I'll ever be able to find another position like it.
- **Jessica:** Oh Sandy, I'm really getting how much you love your job and how worried you are that you'll lose it.
- **Sandy:** Yeeeaaah. I can't believe how stupid I was to tell off my boss when he asked me if I could postpone my vacation till after the project was over. I don't know what I was thinking! I didn't even entertain the idea. I just reacted.

- **Jessica:** Are you maybe feeling some embarrassment and regret because you didn't respond in a way that reflects your thoughtfulness and care?
- **Sandy:** Yeeees! Exactly! I just reacted because I think I was afraid of being taken advantage of again. I'm not used to bosses asking me. I'm used to them telling me so that I either have to listen or leave. I feel so embarrassed.
- **Jessica:** Yeah, I'm getting that embarrassment. And it sounds like in the past your only choices have been to either comply or leave. Is that right?
- **Sandy:** Yes. Thank you so much for hearing me, it really feels good to talk this out.

Notice in this scenario how Jessica either reflected what she was hearing or made empathic guesses about underlying feelings and needs helping Sandy connect more deeply with her own experience. Jessica refrained from giving any advice or suggestions. Sandy was in pain; the last thing she needed was advice. Instead, she needed to be heard, understood, and resonated with. Empathy, over sympathy, helped Sandy delve deeper into herself. When we can empathize and resonate with people in their pain, we give them the gift of being brought deeper into their own experience, heard on a heart level, and resonated with so that they feel accompanied. Ultimately, being with people in their pain is not about solving their experience, it's about being present in it with them. The empathic process also naturally shifts both the listener's and speaker's bodies into a state of connection and safety, which not only feels wonderful but is also health promoting.

People howling in pain or discomfort typically can't hear our words of wisdom. It's possible that after being heard and understood, Sandy might be in a better place to hear advice about her situation. But a word of caution may be helpful here: if we are trying to hear a person's pain in order to give them advice, that's an agenda that the more perceptive among us can sense. Rather than give advice right away, it is much better to wait until the person asks for it. And if we feel urgency around sharing a suggestion or some advice, then at the least, we should hear the person fully, confirm that their need to be heard has been fully met, and only then ask if they are open to hearing our thoughts. In this way, we maintain connection while meeting our needs for care and contribution and their needs for respect and consideration.

When a person engages us in conversation, in essence that person is making a request of us. It is a request for our full attention and complete presence. It's a request to listen. For this reason, it's helpful to realize this so we can check in with ourselves to determine whether listening is something we truly want to do at that moment. If we are going to listen, we want to be "in choice" about it; we don't want to feel obligated to do it at that moment. We want our listening to be a gift we can freely give. The problem with listening to someone when we're really not up for it is that we may begin to feel resentful. And instead of taking responsibility by letting the other person know it's not the best time for us to listen, we judge and blame the other person for talking "too much." The responsibility falls on us to honor our own capacity in the moment and to determine whether we can listen with love at that moment without cost to us and the other person. If listening carries such costs, then letting that person know we care but that we aren't in the best place to listen at the moment will protect everyone's hearts and the health of the relationship. Setting a later time to listen will additionally meet our need for care in the moment and their need for support.

Our resources are finite. On a given day, we only have so much attention, energy, and time to meet our various needs. Using our finite resources within our day to meet as many of our needs as possible is crucial for our health and well-being. So, for example, on a given day, if we spend the majority of our inner resources on work, neglecting our needs for connection, play, exercise, or rest, then our health and well-being will eventually suffer as a result. In fact, learning how to allocate our resources to meet the majority of our needs each day is how we have the strength to sustainably care for and contribute to others.

We have found that being able to create healthy, caring boundaries allows compassionate giving and joyful contribution to flow more effectively. Remember that what can happen when we find ourselves giving beyond our comfort level is a feeling of resentment. The key is to have warm, not harsh, boundaries around your needs, as warm boundaries protect not just our own well-being, but also the health and sustainability of our relationships. With warm boundaries you communicate, "I want to stay in connection with you while doing what works for me and caring about you." Unfortunately, most of us connect boundaries to experiences where we (or others) waited until they were at the end of their rope to react. In that state, boundaries were set with little-to-no warmth and compassion. We want to emphasize that instead, we are talking here about warm boundaries. With warm boundaries it is essential to set them early and not wait until you have experienced more than you can take. This happens when we begin to connect to and discern our internal capacity, along with an intention to care for and connect with another regarding strategies that meet both our needs and theirs.

Alona's growing pains with boundaries

The other day, failing to connect to myself resulted in a disconnection with Matt. Walking into his office, I told him we needed to talk. In hindsight, I would have loved to have noticed my own growing sense of urgency and tightness (both indicative of needs not being met). Instead, I proceeded to tell him that I could not be in charge of Kylee's homeschooling (a recent shift we had made and were still figuring out) and that he needed to be involved. My own tension was transferring to him and he tightly responded, "Okay." This relational tension is common when urgency is felt without connection or clarity. Instead of bringing us together, my strategy was pulling us apart—the last thing I desired at that moment.

My learning was to step back and reconnect with my heart. What I was needing at that moment was understanding and partnership. Connecting to those needs gave me enough resources to have a different conversation. I tried again, "Hey Matt,

I am feeling really anxious and worried about Kylee's homeschool education. I am unclear on how to proceed and really want to make sure she gets the support she needs to be successful. For now, I don't have anything for you to do with regards to Kylee's schooling. However, I would love some empathy for my nervousness as well as reassurance that we are going to figure this out together. Would you be willing to tell me what you are hearing?"

Matt's reflection provided me the support and sense of partnership that I was needing. I knew this intellectually but also felt it in my body as a softening and release of the tightening I had earlier. This was a powerful lesson on the benefit of being present, in a given moment, with my own needs.

Exhaustion (ignoring present needs until they can no longer be overlooked) used to be my indicator that I could not do one more thing. It became very apparent recently that it was not a sustainable strategy. So I have begun working on setting boundaries that serve to protect my time and energy. I no longer want to contribute all that I am doing just because I can. My hope is to strengthen my self-connection to my needs, in a given moment, so that I speak up before I am completely burned out. However, learning to discern what works for me and share it in a way that fosters connection isn't always easy. This is especially so while still in the learning stage. To me, it's like turning your main waterline on after it has been shut off for a while. The faucets begin by sputtering out or spurting out water and slowly adjust to their natural flow. Similarly, when learning a new communication skill, we may miss the mark, stumble into it, or come off too strong until we, too, find our balance. The key is to keep practicing (let the water flow) until it feels natural and becomes habitual.

In the example below, Mary will attempt to engage Todd in a heartfelt conversation. Todd has been feeling very depleted at work these days because of a project deadline and so by the end of his day he's been needing more rest and relaxation than he normally does. Engaging in a deeper emotional conversation is something he currently has little capacity for. However, Todd and Mary are good friends, so he really wants to communicate his care while still holding a clear, warm boundary for himself.

- **Mary:** Hey Todd! How are you?
- **Todd:** Hey Mary! Doing well. It's been a long day, but I can't complain.
- **Mary:** Todd, I have something really important to share with you. I was able to have that conversation with my dad that I was dreading. Remember, the one I asked you for advice about?
- **Todd:** Oh Mary, I'm so happy for—
- **Mary:** (interrupting) You would have been so proud of me! I was able to hold space for both of our needs in the conversation. And we found a way to make our family vacation work for both of us. This is how it happened—
- **Todd:** (interrupting) Mary, excuse me. Can I break in for a second? I am feeling really torn at the moment. A part of me would love to sit on this bench and listen to every detail. Another part of me is absolutely run down after work today and I'm finding myself really needing some down time. I really do want to hear about your conversation. Could we talk about it this weekend when our families get together?
- **Mary:** Oh… I'm sorry… you mentioned wanting to know about it as soon as it happened, and I was so excited to tell you. I didn't mean for it to weigh you down or drain you.
- **Todd:** You're absolutely right, I do want to know. And I look forward to hearing all about it. I just want to be in a place to really enjoy the details and I know that if we got into it now, I wouldn't be able to appreciate it as much.
- **Mary:** Don't worry about it, Todd, I get it.
- **Todd:** But I just want to make sure it works for you to wait until this weekend?

- **Mary:** I mean you know how it is with our kids and all the requests. We'd be lucky to get a few sentences in before the waterfall of interruptions begins.
- **Todd:** True. And I want to hear you without interruptions. What about during lunch tomorrow? Are you free for lunch?
- **Mary:** I am.
- **Todd:** Would you enjoy sharing with me then?
- **Mary:** Absolutely! Let's do it.

In this example, when Mary approached Todd with her request for attention and a listening ear, Todd had two very real parts of himself come up. One part knew he really needed rest and relaxation. Another part wanted to care for and contribute to his friend. Knowing that his needs for rest and relaxation were greater at that moment, he used a warm boundary. When Mary began her story, Todd kindly interrupted her. He then communicated the truth of his present state. That he really wanted to listen but also needed some time to himself. This is the essence of a warm boundary. It's protecting what is most alive in us at the moment, while still communicating our care. In this case, it was meeting a need for care while saying "no" to a request for immediate attention, in order to meet a more pressing need for rest. And to meet his need for care, Todd made sure to find another time that worked for both of them, for Mary to share her story.

Warm boundaries are more about how we intend to protect our own needs or resources—what we'll do or choose not to do—than about what others do. Additionally, warm boundaries are flexible depending on what our needs and the other person's are. Let's use the example above with a slight adjustment. Imagine that Mary came to Tom, deeply distressed because her father was severely injured in a car accident. Although Tom's need for rest and relaxation is great, after hearing from Mary, his need to care for her would become even greater. Thus, he would no longer feel inclined to have a boundary around his need for rest. It's important to remember that warm boundaries are needs-based, not rules-based, giving us the flexibility to protect what is most precious to us at the present moment.

Similar to warm boundaries, life-serving agreements are also meant to protect needs and resources in caring ways. However, as we'll see, these agreements require the collaboration and cooperation of others to make them work. Both agreements and warm boundaries are meant to protect needs and resources in a way that preserves care and harmony. The main difference, however, is that boundaries are about us as individuals, while agreements require a level of collaboration and cooperation for them to work. Agreements are therefore about what *we* are going to do. It becomes clear that an agreement would be helpful when there's a recurring situation that tends to leave someone's needs unmet. The spirit behind an agreement is to find a strategy of handling that recurring situation that works for both people involved.

The first step is to determine what needs are being met by what's happening and what needs are not being met. It is crucial to first become clear on and connect around each person's needs before trying to figure out a strategy. Otherwise, we run the risk of simply tipping the scales in the other direction. An agreement reached without taking this prior step wouldn't be a true life-serving agreement. It's very important to place all the needs on the table, ideally in a warm, respectful, and non-judgmental way. When people focus on the quality of connection instead of the strategies or ideas around what to do, then through that quality of connection the most caring and effective strategies will arise.

Alona's Story

While Matt was traveling, he was on a video call with Jordan. In the middle of the conversation, she wanted to ask Kylee, who was in another room, a question. Her strategy was to yell as loud as she could from her chair, hoping that Kylee could hear her. While on the video call, Matt explained that his ears were hurting from the yelling and requested that she please get up and go into Kylee's room to get her question answered. She was faced with two choices, none of which she liked. She didn't want to get up and she cared about the impact of the yelling on Matt's ears, while still really wanting her question answered. Jordan took a pause and then tended to the quality of the connection by checking in with Matt. She asked, "Dad, so your need is to not hear yelling?" He responded, "Yes, that's correct. So would you please get up and go into the other room?" As you can see, Matt was focused on the strategy of her getting up, which she didn't want to do. She then smiled and said, "I got it, Dad." Jordan proceeded to put the video call on mute while she repeated her question to Kylee. In this manner, both Matt and Jordan were able to meet their needs. I didn't even think of muting the video call, but because Jordan paused to focus on the quality of connection, more strategies became available to her.

Another potential hang-up when trying to find life-serving agreements is getting caught up around what is fair. Fairness is tricky, since everyone typically wants to be in a relationship where there's a sense of mutuality, where both people matter and one person's needs don't eclipse the other's. It's also true, however, that sometimes one person has a greater need for something. One partner may have greater needs for affection and attention than his/her partner does in a given moment. This is neither bad nor good, right or wrong. It just is. We could get caught up arguing over how one person's need for affection and attention is too much, or the other person's need is too little, leading us directly into disconnection. To preserve care and harmony in the relationship, we can explore additional strategies, including setting warm boundaries and creating agreements that aim to meet needs for both partners.

Consider the following example: Nancy and Carol are life partners. Since their jobs became remote about a month ago, they've been working from the living room of their small apartment. Nancy's job requires a couple of zoom meetings a day that require privacy. But Nancy doesn't like doing her zoom meetings in the bedroom. Up until last week, Carol has been willing to relocate into their bedroom while Nancy had her zoom meetings in the living room. However, since her workload has increased, Carol has been noticing some resentment coming up over being the one to move into the bedroom. The issue came to a head when Carol found herself moving into their bedroom around 6 pm to finish her work so that Nancy could watch her favorite TV show in the living room. Watching that show is something they used to do together before Carol's workload increased. Below is an example of the two women trying to work out a life-serving agreement.

Example of a Life Serving Agreement

- **Nancy:** Carol, honey, I'm about to watch my show. Just want to give you a heads up.
- **Carol:** (grumbling) Okay, I'll head to the bedroom.
- **Nancy:** I'm getting the sense that you're not happy. What's up?
- **Carol:** Honestly, I think all this moving back and forth is beginning to take a toll on me. The story I'm telling myself is that I'm doing it just for you—it's all about you and what you want. And I'm beginning to feel resentful and like I don't really matter here.
- **Nancy:** I'm so glad we're talking about this. I could tell that you've been a little quieter, but I thought it was just the stress of the extra work. I'd love to figure out how to make this work!
- **Carol:** Before we move to strategies, I'd like to have some more empathy around my discomfort. I think I'd like some assurance that you know why I might be feeling the way that I am. Could you tell me back what you heard me say earlier?
- **Nancy:** Sure. I heard you say that the story you're telling yourself is that it's all about accommodating what works for me. And that you'd really like the sense that I'm giving to this relationship as much as you are. That you matter too. Did I get it?
- **Carol:** Yes, thank you. And I think I'd like a greater sense that we're in this together. Even with your show. We used to watch it together. Now you're watching without me, and I feel sad.
- **Nancy:** I'm hearing that there's sadness that I am watching the show without you and that you'd like to have a greater sense of togetherness, maybe even some more partnership?
- **Carol:** Yes. Thank you. I appreciate the empathy.

- **Nancy:** If it's okay with you, before we move to strategies, I'd like to know again why it doesn't work for you to move into our bedroom with your laptop for your zoom meetings.
- **Carol:** Sure, I feel embarrassed that my bosses and co-workers will see our bed in the background. I think it's around my need for an identity that is professional. I also think I am needing belonging and acceptance from my peers. They all have home offices. I already feel slightly uncomfortable with our kitchen as the background.
- **Nancy:** I can totally appreciate your need for acceptance, belonging, and professionalism. I think I have a strategy that might work. Are you open to hearing it? (Notice how Nancy asked if Carol was ready to shift from empathy to strategizing)
- **Carol:** Sure!
- **Nancy:** What if we put our bed on the opposite side of the room? We could then set up a table and chair next to the window. That way you can do your zooms from the bedroom without anyone seeing the bed. What do you think?
- **Carol:** I think it's absolutely worth a try.
- **Nancy:** Now, what about my TV show? You mentioned feeling bad that I am watching it without you and that you'd like a greater sense of togetherness.
- **Carol:** Well, would you be willing to record the show so that we could watch it after I finish my work?
- **Nancy:** Yes, love. We can give that a try too.

Notice from this example how tending to the quality of connection first and foremost cultivated good will and care rather than defensiveness, leading to an abundance of strategies instead of a sense of scarcity. Furthermore, getting clear on the needs at stake helped to create a strategy that could potentially work for both women. This is not to say that their strategy will work out. It could be that their neighbor's TV is against the shared wall of Nancy and Carol's bedroom, and often during the time of Nancy's meetings, the neighbor's TV is on at a volume that is too disruptive. If that were the case, it would just mean that the two women would go back to the drawing board to try to find another strategy that might work for both.

Life-serving agreements are experiments that we agree to try. In other words, just because you made an agreement doesn't mean it can't be changed. If the agreement turns out not to work because there are unmet needs still surfacing for one or more individuals, then everyone agrees to come back to the table and tend to the quality of connection, making space for new strategies to come and experiment with. This is different than simply not following through with your agreement because it doesn't work for you, as that would not meet the need for care for another person. Similarly, continuing with an agreement that turns out not to work for you doesn't meet the need for self-care. Life-serving agreements meet needs for care for everyone. The key is to remember that they are dynamic and can shift, as long as we stay tightly connected to the needs of everyone involved rather than to a specific strategy with which to meet those needs.

Our Story

Matt agreed to pick the kids up from school every day, but after a couple of weeks noted that he was tired. A conventional agreement would force him to continue with his commitment, resulting in building resentment and growing depletion over time. A life-serving agreement makes space to create a quality of connection with Alona around caring for her needs for predictability and support as well as Matt's needs for self-care and support. Having a warm, caring quality of connection where all needs are valued and each person's capacity is clarified allows additional strategies to arise and be experimented with. Interestingly, in having that quality of connection, Matt met a need for appreciation he wasn't previously aware he had. Additionally, he realized how valuable his contribution was for Alona. Knowing how his actions contributed, along with a sense of appreciation, resulted in an internal shift to where Matt was willingly to continue to pick up the kids. However, now the energy fueling him was completely different, without resentment, coming from choice and full of a sense of satisfaction.

Like warm boundaries, agreements are flexible and are by no means set in stone. They can be adapted as often as needed to preserve care and harmony. Developing a life-serving agreement isn't about coming up with rules for each person to keep. The intention is to keep the relationship connective and warm by working together. It's an ongoing "togetherness project" where the guidelines shift based upon who needs what. The key, as introduced in the beginning of the chapter, is to share authentically and vulnerably; that's what keeps the connection rich and meaningful. Remember, if we want our conversations with others to have emotional depth, then communicating from the heart is essential. And we do this when we tell others what we value or need at a given moment, how we feel, and what we experience when our needs or values are met or unmet.

At WeHeal, we focus on the quality of connection first and foremost with children as well. Through this quality of connection, we believe all needs become apparent, and mutually satisfying strategies can emerge. Some people may erroneously interpret this as "permissive" parenting. We strongly believe it is just the opposite. In fact, this needs-based consciousness in parenting ensures you will be aware of your needs and be able to meet those needs *more* effectively. "Power-over," or authoritarian, parenting reactively meets the most pressing parent's need in the moment, usually relief and ease over kindness, care, and respect. And this often comes at the expense of the child's needs. On the other end of the spectrum, "permissive parenting" meets the children's needs at the expense of the parent's needs. The third option, "power-with parenting," cares for the parent's needs and the children's needs, and this is the type of parenting we strive for.

For example, if you are needing peace and quiet, you may reactively demand that your child be quiet. That is power-over parenting. Suppressing your needs, while allowing the child to do whatever they want, is permissive parenting. There is a third way, power-with parenting, where you create a quality of connection with your child to put both of your needs on the table. Once that quality of connection is created, there is a trust that you can collaborate on strategies that could work for both of you. No one needs to submit (compromise or "give in") or rebel (fight, argue, or shut down). Instead, there arises an interdependent relationship in which there is a desire to care about and contribute to one another—along with a trust that together, you will find solutions that work for all.

When you simply tell your child to stop doing something, without first connecting to their needs, you essentially communicate that their needs don't matter. This contributes to three key needs that often go chronically unmet in children, resulting in the toxic submit-rebel paradigm that most parents fall into. Those three needs are their need to be heard, to have choice, and to trust that their needs matter. When children believe that they don't have choice and that their needs don't matter, they believe they either need to submit to their parents or rebel against them. When kids are young and less powerful, they often submit; however, when they move into their teenage years and discover more power and agency, they shift over to rebellion. Submission and rebellion are, in fact, two sides of the same disconnected coin.

In our family, anytime we have a sense that our children are submitting, we see a red flag to tend to the connection. We do this not only because we want their needs to matter and for them to have choice, but because the more they submit as younger children, the more likely it is that they will rebel as older children. If you don't tend to connection, you induce disconnection. As a result, every time we sense submission, we see not only pain and disconnection in the moment but even greater pain and disconnection in the future. Instead, we want to build trust with our children that we value connection more than getting our way. It is this trust that is going to help determine whether teenagers and adult children value and trust the relationship with their parents.

Sure, teenagers may desire to build their independence, but they don't want to rebel and disconnect from their parents. Most teenagers with whom we have worked long for a deeper connection with their parents. Sadly, they simply don't know how to achieve that, nor do they trust that their parents want it. Their rebellion is a tragic strategy to get some of their needs met when they see the alternative as suppressing their needs to maintain a relationship with their parents. We say *some* of their needs because one of their needs is to be connected with their family. The need to belong is a biological imperative, but that need will be sacrificed if their autonomy and self-connection are threatened.

Don't make your children choose between connection and autonomy! Instead, focus on tending to the quality of connection between you and your children whenever possible. We do this by asking our children to always tell us when they hear "bossiness" (a term little children understand) or "demands" (the implication that there will be some emotional or physical consequence if they don't do what is asked), as that provides an opportunity to check inside and "redo" the interaction in an effort to support the quality of connection first and foremost. Although it may be more "efficient" to get your way in the short term by making demands and supporting the power-over paradigm with submission, if you are invested in a long-term connection with your children, then power-with parenting is the sure bet.

Failing to build trust and care for each other is detrimental not only to the children but also to the parents. When resourced, parents can easily see how power-with parenting feels more natural and congruent with their internal values, but when under-resourced, as most parents often are, it is easy to lose sight of this. The immediate relief experienced with power-over parenting comes at great cost. What's more, it is hard to see that cost in the reactive moment when old, habitual parenting strategies are taking over. Through patience, self-compassion, and dedication to personal growth, parenting can be different.

Marshall Rosenberg used to say that we need to answer two questions to be effective parents: one, what do we want our children to do; and two, what do we want the reason to be behind what they do? By learning to value the quality of connection between you and your children, you will ensure that *all* needs are cared for, which will ensure a strong quality of connection now, through the teenage years, and beyond. What's more, it's never too late to start rebuilding that trust by contributing to your children's needs to be heard, to have choice, and to matter!

As parents, we have two major needs: peace of mind that our children will be okay, and contribution to their well-being. Effective parenting is not about spending the correct amount of time together or doing any specific activity together; rather, it is about how you show up. P.L.A.E., or **Presence, Loving Attention, and Empathy** are the keys to supporting your child's authentic self to come alive and be accepted. When not sure what to do, be emotionally present, provide loving and caring attention, and empathize with whatever is alive in them. It is not complicated, but it also isn't easy, as you have to manage your own needs and reactivity, do your own growth work through your pain and wounding, and still make room for others... all at the same time! So with compassion and clear intention, it is not about getting it "right" with your children all of the time; rather, it is a mindset in which you acknowledge mistakes, repair them, and do your best the next time around. With this intention as your guide, connection will always be within your grasp! If parents could simply P.L.A.E. ("play") with their children, then we believe this world would be a much better place for both children and parents.

Missing the mark with empathy—if they are still mad, you didn't get it

Alona's story

Kylee was upset with her sister for pointing out a pimple she had on her face and saying that it was gross. Realizing right away that she may have stimulated pain in her sister, Jordan apologized. Yet Kylee was still furious and adamant about receiving an apology in a very specific way. This created a lot of confusion, especially for Jordan, who couldn't understand why her apology was not enough. She clearly stated that she did not mean to hurt Kylee's feelings and wished she had never said it. Jordan even empathized with how bad Kylee was feeling. Why

Kylee remained so angry wasn't clear to me, either. A part of me was thinking, "Hey kid, enough! Get over yourself already. She already apologized and shared her regret so why are you still making such a big deal out of this?" Thankfully, I recognized my judgments, therefore keeping them in my own head, and realized how they would impact Kylee, particularly signaling to her anger was "wrong" and should be suppressed in the future. But I was noticeably tighter than I would have liked to be; I was feeling less open and more contracted.

In that state, I tried to give Kylee empathy. As we discussed, true empathy is being present with another without an agenda of your own. I was giving Kylee empathy while really wanting her to stop being upset. In short, it was not real empathy. At one point, I realized we were going nowhere and asked for a pause. Thinking about the situation, I remembered that EVERYTHING we do is to meet a need. In other words, Kylee's continued upset was meeting some need. It became clear then that we hadn't tapped into the underlying need. She was still angry because we didn't fully understand her. Realizing this, I was able to let go of my own agenda and shift my attention towards Kylee.

Focusing completely on Kylee brought to my awareness the harsh judge that lives in her head. Imagining what it might be saying to her, I shared out loud some empathy guesses around her pain and anger. Although she didn't respond, I could see her begin to soften. Eventually I got to a guess around embarrassment and shame. I suggested that her own judge was mirroring Jordan's words, but instead of "the pimple is gross," it was screaming "you are gross!" Hearing this, she completely softened and a tear fell from her eye. It turned out that Kylee needed empathy for her internal judge and all the pain it stimulated. Being with Kylee as she experienced this pain allowed her to feel accompanied. Jordan, who was present through this exploration, was also able to hold that space. Kylee felt she was not alone; she didn't have to hold all that pain by herself. With that empathic presence and connection, she found the peace and acceptance she needed.

The takeaway for me was that when someone perseverates on an issue, not letting it go well beyond your tolerance or understanding, there is always a reason. Often, more empathy and understanding are needed. This is an invitation to dive deeper with that person as you support a greater connection and more complete healing.

CHAPTER 14

Work

Pillar 7

"Too many of us are not living our dreams
because we are living our fears."

—LES BROWN

M OST OF US IN OUR WESTERN culture spend some portion of our
week relating to people we work with or for, either remotely or
in person. In fact, a good number of us spend more time in our work
relationships than in any other relationships. It thus becomes a worthwhile goal to make whatever time we spend at work as enjoyable and
satisfying as possible.

Sadly, many feel isolated in their work environment, while others
don't feel emotionally comfortable or even safe. As a result, we suppress
or deny a part of ourselves to get by. We refer to this as being in a state
of artificial harmony. Over time, being in this state takes a toll on us.
What's more, suppressing our authentic selves while at work is interpreted by our bodies as a threat. As you are now aware, suppression
implies threat, and threat stimulates a physiological state of inflammation and other changes that, when permitted to exist chronically, can
wreak havoc on our health. So, if our health and happiness are a priority, it behooves us to adopt a particular mindset at work that improves
our resourcing and connection skills and allows us to eliminate the
suppression that signals threat to our bodies.

While we can't control how others show up and relate to us on the
job, there are concrete ways to empower and make life better for our-

selves. In doing so, we increase our chances of cooperation, flow, and efficiency, regardless of whether we are the employer or the employee. Our focus will always be on what we can control: our behavior and reactions, not other people's actions. What you will find is that when you change how you show up and react, the people around you will change as a result. This impact is unavoidable but it cannot be your goal; instead, think of it as a welcome side effect.

Improving our experience at work starts with the recognition that we have needs and that meeting them is crucial. In fact, unless our physical and emotional needs are met regularly, we will not be able to operate at our best.

SOME COMMON NEEDS	
Acceptance/Belonging	Kindness
Affection/Care	Learning
Appreciation	Mourning
Autonomy/Choice	Movement
Celebration	Mutuality
Challenge	Nourishment
Clarity	Nurturing
Comfort	Order
Compassion	Partnership
Competence	Peace
Consideration	Play
Contribution	Purpose/Meaning
Dignity	Reassurance
Ease	Relief
Fairness	Respect
Friendship	Rest

Growth	Safety
Health	Security
Honesty	Support
Hope	To be Heard
Independence	To Matter
Integrity	Trust
Joy	Understanding

Very few of us meet most of our needs through our line of work. For some, work deeply meets needs for meaning and purpose. These are the folks who'd continue to do what they're doing even if they won the lottery. For others, work may meet needs for connection, stimulation, discovery, engagement, and challenge, but not meaning or purpose. And then there are those who are only meeting their need for financial security and survival. Whatever our situation may be, it's important that we still make it a priority to identify and try to meet needs in other ways if they aren't being met through our work.

For example, those who are unable to meet needs for meaning and purpose with their work (those working simply to earn money for food and shelter) can choose to meet their need to contribute to society outside of their work.

Now this isn't to say that another line of work, another position in one's company, or an altogether different business venture may not meet more of our needs. But unless we truly learn what it takes to meet our own needs, a vocational move might just land us in a position where some needs are met more fully, but others much less. We may find ourselves hopping from business to business or from job to job, not realizing the extent to which our work can truly satisfy us.

With a needs-based awareness, you can find great satisfaction in many jobs. Matt has fond memories of jobs that were not very fun or exciting but the people he worked with made work enjoyable, and he experienced some wonderful connections. He also had other jobs that seemed promising on paper yet turned out to be miserable because the community and work environment were unbearable. In other words, it's less about the job and more about the needs. For example, if there are deeper, core personal needs (e.g., self-care, love, play, celebration of life) that are out of balance, then until these needs are met, you may not find satisfaction from any job. It is therefore important to note that regardless of the job, some degree of resourcing will always be necessary. Accordingly, knowing ourselves (and our needs) better, and learning how to resource ourselves wherever we are at in life, puts us in the best position to determine whether a vocational move is in our best interest or not.

A resource is anything that can be used to meet a need. Resourcing ourselves means simply meeting our needs with what we have available to us. We have internal and external resources to choose from.

Let's start by considering external resources, which usually fall into three categories: people, places, or things. For example, friendships can be a tremendous resource for us. Spending time with a friend can meet needs for connection, closeness, fun, stimulation, warmth, joy, attention, affection, care, and more. Literature, music, and art are also resources meeting needs for aliveness, stimulation, inspiration, beauty, and celebration. Nature can be considered another resource. For instance, a park, nature trail, or beach can meet needs for rest, beauty, health, inspiration, transcendence, discovery, and more. Education in the form of recreational or vocational classes or workshops can meet needs for learning, growth, discovery, challenge, efficiency, and progress. Even on a level of survival, our home is a resource, as it meets needs for shelter and comfort. Food and water meet our needs for nutrition and hydration.

It's imperative to find what needs of ours aren't being met through work and find the resources we have available to us to meet those needs off the job. For example, let's say our job isn't providing us opportunities for growth, challenge, or learning. We could meet those needs outside of work with hobbies. Learning a foreign language, a martial art, or ballroom dance could be ways to meet those needs. If finances preclude these options, access to a public library provides a free resource. Reading itself may invite a new hobby into our lives, or simply allow us to enjoy literary classics. Different forms of exercise such as walking, running, calisthenic training, aerobics, or yoga may be options, too. And since we all have to eat, improving upon our cooking or baking skills can be both practical and pleasurable. All of these strategies have the potential to meet needs for challenge, growth, and learning and can be routinely done when time allows and with a minimal outlay of money to start and maintain. The key is that once our needs have been identified, multiple strategies will exist to meet them. Our job is to find the ones that work best for us.

Let's now consider internal resources. An image comes to mind of a weary traveler, thirsty and hot, crossing a desert. One step after the other, she lumbers through the sand, her feet sinking with each step. She's aching to quench her thirst and get relief from the blazing heat. At the start of her journey, she had found a backpack full of stuff. Without opening it up, she had thrown it on her back, thinking that at some point it could come in handy. All the while, she failed to discover that the backpack contained a canteen of water, a hat, a pair of sunglasses, dried fruits and nuts, and a map showing a paved route through the sands—resources that would have made her journey more sustainable and much less burdensome. But what is unrealized is unutilized.

Like the weary traveler, many of us are not aware of the resources we already possess internally. Taking stock of our internal resources is important in order to make our journey more sustainable and enjoyable. Internal resources include our knowledge, skills, abilities, beliefs, and even our very attention. The simple act of taking stock will meet needs in and of itself, such as needs for inspiration, hope, and clarity. And where you put your attention matters, as that is often what will manifest. In other words, if you put your intention on needs, then you will be much more likely to meet them.

The point of taking stock of our own internal resources, after all, is to determine how we can best use our knowledge, skills, and abilities to resource ourselves. So ultimately it doesn't matter if you choose to play the guitar or if you just enjoy finger painting. Both can meet the same needs for creativity, challenge, and inspiration.

The ability to make requests is an internal resource with the potential to grant us access to resources we don't possess. As we've evolved to meet many of our needs in community with other people, cooperation and resource sharing with others is essential to our well-being. And yet, for many reasons, we may be hesitant to ask others for what we want or need. Maybe we're too embarrassed to admit that we have certain needs, such as needing a loan or needing help with marital issues. Maybe we're afraid that if we admit that we need something, it could be used against us. Perhaps we avoid making requests for fear that we'll be obliged to return the favor in some way that we won't feel free to say "no" to. Or maybe we're afraid to hear a "no" because we'll internalize it as rejection and that would be too crushing for us to handle. There's no denying that some of these fears may be legitimate; we may have good reasons for not asking people for help based on our past experience.

At the same time, many of us have room to grow in making requests of others, especially if we want to live in a state of Life Is Wonderful. All too often, we miss out on opportunities to resource ourselves for reasons that are worth working through. Fear derived from past experience, along with stories of what we imagine will happen, lead us to a perpetual state of not meeting our needs. Yet stories are just that— stories. As we have no idea what will happen in the present moment, holding onto stories is the surest way to repeat past patterns.

How can we develop our ability to make requests and let go of our stories? Begin with identifying the fears or aversions around asking. Next, decide whether the rationale is truly worth the cost of not getting our needs met that way. For example, maybe you have a fear that your request for help will be rejected, ignored, or denied. Until you ask, you have no idea what the response will be. Just because it has been a "no" in the past doesn't mean it will be so in the present. Another way to develop this resource is by recognizing that everyone, to varying degrees, has a need to care for and contribute to others. Not only are these needs universal, but regularly meeting the needs to care and contribute to others is necessary for our own well-being.

Exercise

Try thinking of something you would like to ask for, but don't because you fear another's reaction. Instead of defaulting to not asking, take a moment to imagine what the worst reaction could be. Now ask yourself, what could you do to empathize with that reaction? This is where your power lies. You can't control another person's reaction, but you can control how you respond to their reaction. For example, let's say you were afraid to ask your boss to review something you wrote because you are worried she will say that she is too busy. Or maybe she wouldn't even say anything, but the look on her face when you ask has you thinking you are inconveniencing her.

That perception stems from a tender need to matter, arising from old childhood wounds (specifically feeling like you didn't matter). Having that awareness around your own need allows you to empathize with your hurt and fear. That, in and of itself, can be so very healing. In addition, knowing that mattering comes up for you, you can also more carefully craft your request as well as prepare yourself for some of the responses you fear. With this in mind, you are no longer asking your partner to review something you wrote and then bracing for a possible yes or no. It is worth noting here that hearing a "yes" may provide temporary relief, but does nothing to heal this dynamic, as it simply kicks the can down the road until the next request. So, instead you can say, "I am nervous to ask you to review what I wrote because when you say that you are too busy, I feel hurt and think I don't matter. Before you tell me whether you can review this or not, could you take a minute to share how you value my work and whether you enjoy contributing to me by reviewing it?"

In this manner, you give your boss a chance to attend to the quality of the connection first and foremost. This allows them to contribute to your needs for care, for your work to matter, and for support without agreeing to review it or not. What matters most here is not whether your boss ends up reviewing your work, but that your needs were named and cared for. After attending to your needs, your boss may still be too busy to review your work. But now, you know it is a measure of their capacity instead of a measure of their care. Because your needs were met, you will more likely be expansive and open to other strategies—maybe your boss can review it later that day or another co-worker can take a pass. Regardless, this situation exemplifies that getting to the needs is at the core of connection and trumps strategy or outcome every time.

Many of us know how good it feels to contribute to the well-being of others, especially when we can connect to the person's need and we're in a place to give freely. Focusing on the opportunity we give to others to tend to the quality of connection (through our requests) may strengthen our resolve and courage—even when those others can't do what we are ultimately asking. Additionally, improving our ability to make requests that will meet more of our needs in the moment (in the example above, we had a need not only for support but also a need for care and mattering), increases our own sense of personal power and agency.

Another powerful internal resource is our attention. Where we place our attention not only has a tremendous impact on our health and well-being, it also has the potential to resolve our conflicts with co-workers with greater efficiency, effectiveness, and care. Say that we have a co-worker—let's call him Ted—who is responsible for importing data into the company server. Our boss needs a project completed by the end of the day, but we can't start our end of the project until Ted's work is complete. Compounding this scenario, we have dinner plans, which we made weeks in advance, with close friends at a new restaurant. And we're now beginning to feel the time crunch. It's already mid-morning and we see Ted drinking coffee and chuckling while reading the funny pages in the breakroom. Since our cubicle is next to the breakroom, we know that this is Ted's second coffee break this morning despite his portion of the job not being finished yet.

Under the circumstances, we likely have thoughts like: *"What the hell is Ted doing? Another coffee break? I'm going to have to stay later today because Lazybones wants more coffee and more time to read the funnies! This is completely unacceptable! He knows I can't start my work until he's done. I might be late for dinner. Or worse, I might miss it."* All the while, we feel agitation, frustration, and annoyance along with concern over missing dinner. Our bodies experience this as a threat with the corresponding physiological shifts that occur as a result. Because we see Ted as a threat, we prepare to defend needs (such as consideration, integrity, ease, and flow) that appear poised to go unmet.

While the details of this example may be unique, this type of work conflict isn't. How we use our resource of attention in cases like this makes a significant difference to our emotional state and the quality of our time at work. For example, if we keep our attention on our judgments about Ted, then feelings of agitation, frustration, and annoyance are likely to continue and deepen. In fact, it's probable that we'll begin to fume with anger and resentment. Likewise, focusing on what's wrong with this situation, what should or shouldn't be the case, or anything along those lines, will prolong this constricted, contracted, and uncomfortable state of mind. However, when we shift our attention to our inner experience, particularly by naming our emotions, we begin to resource ourselves by meeting needs for self-connection, self-regulation, and balance.

A research scientist and professor, Dr. Matthew Lieberman, has found, with the aid of MRI, that activity in the amygdala and limbic regions is diminished when emotions are named.[1] Along these same lines, Dr. Daniel Siegal, a clinical professor of psychiatry at UCLA, coined the phrase, "If you can name it, you can tame it." In other words, simply placing our attention on our emotions and naming them enables our bodies to shift from a state of hyperarousal and threat to a more regulated state of safety. Our stress hormones and chemicals, blood flow, and other inflammatory changes all shift as well. Our emotions let us know whether what we're feeling and perceiving is meeting our needs and values or not. If our perception is that we are meeting our needs or are aligned with our values, we usually experience pleasant feelings or emotions consistent with a physiological state of safety. The opposite is true when what we perceive is interpreted as not meeting our needs or values: we feel unpleasant feelings or emotions which serve as a warning sign that we are experiencing a threat, because when our needs are threatened, our body reacts to defend our survival. By focusing our attention on what our body is communicating and by naming it, the intensity of the message decreases significantly.

Rather than playing into our story or interpretation of the situation, we can focus our attention on what needs of ours are being perceived as unmet and what needs we would like met. In the example with Ted, we would most likely have a need for cooperation, support, efficiency, and consideration. And these needs are compounded by our needs for connection, warmth, play, discovery, and stimulation with our friends later that evening. We can also focus our attention on Ted's needs. Consider that Ted was on his second coffee break. Most likely he's in need of more rest, relaxation, or maybe escape from the tedious nature of his portion of the project. Essentially, Ted is just trying to resource himself. And he's probably needing respect, understanding, and acknowledgment around his decision to resource himself with another coffee break.

Focusing our attention on these motivational forces is not just grounding, it provides clarity and direction if we decide to take action. It doesn't mean we need to agree with Ted's choices and strategies; rather, it just helps cultivate a quality of connection that will be more likely to meet all of our needs. Once our bodies are more regulated by naming the feelings and needs, we would be in a better space to approach Ted with our concern. We could share with Ted how meaningful our plan for the evening is to us and how we're beginning to feel concerned there may not be enough time for us to complete things on our end before our engagement tonight. We can also affirm the importance of taking breaks. Additionally, we could tell him how much time we'll probably need after he's done and whether he thinks our joint efforts will finish the project in time. By presenting the situation in this collaborative way, we increase our likelihood that Ted will be moved by care and compassion to cooperate to the extent that he can.

In contrast, approaching Ted with frustration, annoyance, or resentment would not just lessen the likelihood of his receptivity, it would probably put a strain on the working relationship going forward. Determining the outcome becomes entirely dependent upon how we use our resource of attention. In the example above, how we used our attention helped not just to regulate our system, but to bring clarity and direction to a complicated work dynamic.

In the past, you may have felt there were only two options available to you with regards to work conflicts like the one with Ted. Either you could suppress your needs to maintain artificial harmony with Ted, or you could criticize Ted and sacrifice future harmony and connection. Now we have introduced a third way in which you can be caring for Ted while also sharing vulnerably your concerns and your needs without judgment or criticism. This is what creates the quality of connection that increases the likelihood Ted will naturally care about you and want to contribute and support you to get the work done so you can make your dinner.

Additional ways of regulating our system, at work or at home, are helpful tools to meet needs for peace of mind, rest, and balance. Wherever we may be, we can resource ourselves by simply taking a few moments and placing our attention on our breath. This is different from consciously taking slow and deep breaths. Rather, the instruction would be to gently observe our body while it naturally breathes. When we take time to observe our experience, we are showing our body care. This not only feels wonderful but results in a physiological shift towards the anti-inflammatory state of safety. Take just a few moments to try it now. See if this practice helps increase your sense of calm and peace.

Another strategy to try is placing our attention on any tension, constriction, or contraction that develops in our bodies as we go about our business. When you do so, remember that it is not an effort to make any tension go away, but instead to show your body that you care about how it feels. Again, this creates a sense of safety. Just gently resting our attention on those places is a form of self-connection and self-understanding. Think of tension, constriction, or contraction in the body as a friend in pain that's trying to talk to you about the discomfort. Placing our attention on that tension or constriction with gentleness and kindness is like listening to that friend. And we can give our body that listening ear anytime something comes up. Sometimes we might want to stop what we're doing to listen. But other times we might be able to carry on with our business while also paying attention to the state of our body.

After reading this section on resourcing, you might find yourself lumping together the importance of resourcing ourselves with a need for more self-care. It's here that making a distinction between resourcing and self-care seems relevant. While the two may be aligned, more often in our culture, self-care is associated with the time that we carve out for ourselves in our day or week—that's just for us. It's a time to focus on our health and well-being by doing something kind, nourishing, or good for ourselves. And while this practice is highly encouraged, what is being suggested here is a synergistic strategy for living which is applicable during each moment of our day. Every time we become consciously aware, we can ask ourselves what is needed in that moment for optimal health and well-being and what resources we can mobilize to best meet those needs. In other words, every moment becomes an opportunity for resourcing and self-care.

We can connect, at any moment, with how our work might be resourcing us. Are we talking to a customer or client and meeting needs for connection and stimulation? Are we doing a difficult repair job, meeting needs for challenge and growth? Are we using a body of knowledge that we've accumulated throughout years of experience or study to help someone needing our service or support, meeting needs for competency, care, and contribution? At the very least, is our work meeting our needs for financial sustainability? Connecting to how our work is currently meeting our needs brings a subtle form of appreciation and gratitude that resources us.

Maybe we're beginning to feel fatigue while working. Resourcing ourselves might mean going to the break room for another cup of coffee while skimming through the funny pages again—just as in our example with Ted. In fact, let's imagine that we're in Ted's shoes. We're taking another break and a co-worker approaches us with concern about missing an important dinner engagement. We can tell she has genuine concern about whether she can finish things on her end in time to make her important dinner. And we appreciate how understanding she is about the need to take frequent breaks given the tedious nature of the work. Feeling warmed by her respect and sensing her genuine need for fun and connection, we could resource ourselves by working faster than we normally would to meet our need to care and contribute. In fact, working within a shorter time frame in this situation may even meet our need for efficiency and a challenge.

The question to ask ourselves is: "What can I do to maximize health and well-being at this moment?" When we meet that need, we resource ourselves. Ultimately, caring for ourselves in this way, day after day and moment by moment, allows us to show up at work as the best version of ourselves on a sustainable basis.

Often simply connecting to our needs alone stimulates a sense of peace and safety in our bodies because it is less about meeting all of our needs immediately and more about being aware of their existence. Eliminating artificial harmony in your workplace and replacing it with compassionate authenticity is essential to promote not only long-term work satisfaction but also long-term health. Once we have established the quality of connection that brings needs to the table without judgments and criticisms (which are simply old, tragic, habitual ways of expressing needs), then we can cultivate trust that everyone's needs will be cared for as soon as time and capacity permits. It is within this approach to your work that Life Is Wonderful.

CHAPTER 15

Spirituality

Pillar 8

"Your sacred space is where you can
find yourself over and over again."

—JOSEPH CAMPBELL

THE TERM "SPIRITUAL" CAN mean something substantially different from person to person. For this reason, the word may create more confusion than clarity. Many of us realize that there are aspects of our existence that are both mysterious and miraculous. And yet we want to explore these aspects in a way that's congruent with the principles and patterns we've learned so far. We want a way to be in touch with what is mysterious and miraculous about human existence while not losing touch with what we know from scientific advancements and the practicalities of life—a spirituality that satisfies both our heart and our mind. The orientation of this chapter on spirituality focuses on what is within you as well as how it connects to the world around us, whether miraculous, scientific, or both. How we relate to our own unique experiences and the world around us can either bring about well-being or deep suffering.

The encouragement to live life in the present moment is a common theme in many spiritual teachings. In fact, it's talked about so often that the significance of what it points to is sometimes lost. What "present moment" teachings can bring up for some is discouragement over how often we fail to live there. The urging to live life in the present moment can almost feel like a request to jump much higher than we can. Many of us are all too accustomed to operating throughout our day in a disconnected state, lost in our thoughts. Yet it's undeniable that when we're attuned to our bodies and to what we're doing in the present moment, we often experience a wholeness that's hard to put into words. For example, consider how alive we can feel to just "be" in a moment, connecting to our breath, the space around us, and what we might be feeling at the time, letting go of any thoughts that arise, not having anything that must get done. Or consider what it feels like to savor our food, thoroughly enjoying one bite at a time to connect with the flavors, textures, and full sensation of it all.

You are probably thinking you don't have time for this because you're not a monk in a monastery. And quite possibly, the above examples of present moment engagement and body-mind connection may be off-putting to you since the pace it requires seems incompatible with the demands of actual life. Maybe you're a parent of little ones who require constant supervision just to keep them safe. You might be thinking of how often you find yourself running to the next room, not walking. Or maybe you're a business owner doing everything you can to keep your operation afloat for the sake of your family or employees. Let's face it: taking the time to taste your food isn't a priority. You give food a few chews before swallowing, good enough to prevent choking while planning out your next advertising campaign.

This is the case for most of us. We move throughout our days disconnected from our bodies, going from one task to another, thinking about our next task while we complete our current one. Even when we stop to take a breather, our bodies often just sit vacantly while our attention focuses on the thoughts rushing through our minds. In these moments, we may have a lingering sense that something precious is slipping through our fingers. This is where mindfulness comes in—a space within which we understand, without judgment or criticism, that we are doing our very best in every moment to try to meet our needs. Practicing mindfulness helps us to stay connected to our bodies so that we can fully experience, without shame, blame, or judgment, what it feels like (and how it impacts us) to be lost in thought. It offers us a tool to observe our experiences in a way that we can truly learn from them.

Many of us have attempted to make lifestyle changes by shaming, guilting, or judging ourselves into what we think is a better way to live. We tell ourselves that we *should* be more present. We *should* be more mindful. We *should* finally start that meditation practice. And when we tell ourselves that we *should* do anything, we are trying to get ourselves to do something without really honoring where we are at and why we are doing what we are currently doing. The reason that many of us are not enjoying a more self-connected and present-centered existence is that we haven't known and experienced it as the best way to meet our needs—nor, perhaps, do we believe that it is. We haven't developed the inner trust that we can have both self-connection and presence *with* efficiency and productivity. For a shift to take place, we need to experience both sides of the coin simultaneously, without self-imposed pressure or self-critical judgments.

If we want to enjoy more of what the present moment offers to us, bringing in mindfulness—a non-judgmental awareness of our experience—can help. We can't convince ourselves that something is better for us before we have experienced, again and again, that it's truly a better way. Mindfulness allows our system to do that by supporting discovery and discernment of what truly contributes to our well-being and what doesn't.

In contrast, guilt and shame, as well as judgments like *should* and *ought,* all get in the way of that organic process. As counterintuitive as it sounds, there is benefit to acknowledging these tragic strategies. In doing so, we give attention to what we are doing to meet our needs, even if it is at cost to other needs. We give our mind the space and the freedom to discover if what we're doing truly is the best way to meet the majority of our needs. When we shame, guilt, or *should* ourselves (tragic strategies intended to let us know that we are not in integrity with our values), there's a part of us that digs its heels in and resists change. In psychology, this is called reactance. That part of us doesn't want to be told what to do, doesn't want to be forced or coerced by guilt or shame. But if we can acknowledge, and even appreciate, that we are doing our very best, even if it involves tragic strategies, we avoid inner resistance. In essence, we honor and respect our capacity for personal growth and development in a given moment. To the part of us that truly wants to grow and heal, we allow the opportunity to explore other ways to meet the same needs without cost to our health and well-being.

Connecting to ourselves in the present moment may result in subtle levels of unease, tension, and restlessness. In fact, sometimes these feelings are not so subtle and may even be very uncomfortable. We begin to attempt to fix our feelings by guessing that if only we were more compassionate, wise, warm, evolved, grounded, or maybe more financially secure or successful, we'd have greater ease in the present moment—we'd have more peace. Peace in the present moment becomes something we mistakenly work toward by bettering ourselves. In other words, *once I'm better, my present moment will be better*. But part of us already knows it doesn't make a difference how long we work on ourselves or how many things we secure or accomplish. Truly resting in the present moment isn't a result of doing, it's a matter of being. To find rest in the present moment requires us to meet ourselves where and as we are.

Spiritual practice is, therefore, not about changing our emotional experiences or making them better. It's about letting go of what we think the present moment should be like and beginning to accept and receive our moment as it is. Levels of resistance and reactivity are almost always present in our bodies, even if on a subtle level. This is normal and natural. After all, our species has survived over hundreds of thousands of years because our baseline reactivity has allowed us to react to and neutralize threats. The process of acceptance begins as we attempt to relax our resistance. By slowly realizing that our experiences are neither bad nor good, right nor wrong, we can move from judgment to curiosity around them. Believing an experience must be either bad/good or wrong/right, we force our bodies to identify the experience as either a threat or a sign of safety and succumb to the shifting physiology associated with those two states.

Every conscious moment in our life has a qualitative flavor. Right now, in this moment, your experience has distinct qualities. You have certain bodily sensations, a particular mood, maybe certain feelings. Most likely, you find yourself in an environment replete with colors, sounds, and perhaps smells (whether you are aware of them or not).

All of these make up our present moment experience. Whatever the flavor of our current mood, bodily sensations, emotions, feelings, or thoughts, the practice is to acknowledge them with understanding and curiosity over resistance and reactivity.

We are not suggesting that we *like* everything we experience. That would lack integrity and honesty. But bringing curiosity and understanding to our reactivity helps us be more at peace with whatever arises in our present. At the heart of this practice rests the process of relaxing our resistance to our triggered states. What's the significance of this practice? Why are we shifting from *doing* to *being*, from resisting to accepting? The Dalai Lama said, "There are only two days in the year that nothing can be done. One is called Yesterday and the other is called Tomorrow. Today is the right day to love, believe, do, and mostly live." Living in Today, in this moment, is essentially what we have.

All the same, what can we do when we don't like who we are or what we are experiencing at a given moment? When we feel in some way out of sorts, unfocused, constricted, dull, jittery, or pained? It comes down to this: Can we simply breathe with our present moment? Can we hold our experience, with warmth and intentionality, and breathe? Instead of thinking about whether you agree with these words or not, try breathing with your current mood, sensations, emotions, and thoughts. Let them all be there. Just breathe. This isn't about changing anything. Just experiment and breathe with your current experience for as long as it feels good to you. Try it right now.

What happens when we're able to simply breathe with our experience, whatever it might be, is that our brain begins to tell us that we're safe. That we can make it. If we can consciously breathe, then we can find a way to be in this moment and accept it. And the message that slowly begins to register within us is that we can accept ourselves regardless of whatever experience we're having. We can hold ourselves with warmth and understanding no matter what. Robert Gonzales, a certified trainer in Nonviolent Communication, referred to this process as radical relaxation and unconditional acceptance. He made the point that what transforms us is our relationship to the experience, not the experience itself.

Radically relaxing into our emotional experiences and our present moments doesn't equate to resignation to our current life circumstances or relationships. We can still work to change what we don't like. The difference is that we approach things much differently. When we are at peace with our own experience, we are more likely to show up with more care, respect, and collaboration. Ultimately our shift supports empowerment; not only can we change our circumstances, but now we can do so from a more expansive place.

There are times when breathing with, and relaxing around, a particular emotional experience is what our system most needs. That is particularly true when we find ourselves uncomfortable, disconnected from our bodies, or resisting the moment. If, however, we have a strong emotional charge based on a particularly challenging story about a situation or experience, relating to ourselves with words may be a better approach. In her book, *Your Resonant Self*, Sarah Peyton introduces the concept of resonant language. She writes, *"This type of language includes wondering about and naming emotion; dreams, longings, and needs; body sensations; and fresh metaphor, visual imagery, and poetry."*[1] Using resonant language (or what we call self-empathy) to accompany ourselves around emotional experiences brings more than just acceptance; it brings warmth, self-understanding, self-compassion, and a very real sense of accompaniment. All of these together provide a safe space to release repression and suppression and instead open ourselves up to reflection and processing. Consider the example below about an experience involving a father and his teenage son. Notice how the father is simply accompanying himself in his experience, not in an effort to change anything or fix anything but just to be with his emotions and experience:

Self-Resonance or Self-Empathy with a Challenging Experience

(Dad's inner voice with self-empathy language)

Do you feel a sadness and sense of loss when you think of your connection to your boy? Missing the days when you and he were able to connect with more ease and warmth? The days when you had something that you both shared, enjoyed, and looked forward to together? Are you just exhausted from negotiating on so many levels and is your heart weary and longing for ease and escape? Would you like some acknowledgment of how difficult a challenge this experience is for you—how each day seems to offer a new way to let go of how you think he should be or how life should go? Do you wish you could just push a button to let go of all your painful expectations, so they'd release off your body like lead weights?

Would you like some acknowledgment of your sadness and disappointment when you relate to him in ways that don't meet your own needs for compassion and care? Do you wish you could contribute to his development more than you are?

Self-empathy happens when a part of us steps outside of our current experience and begins to relate to that experience as a "witness" with resonant language. In the above example, a warm, welcoming "witness" is resonating with a recurring experience this father is having with his son. We can do this with any experience we have. When it comes to more challenging emotional experiences, it's important to note that self-resonance doesn't take away our uncomfortable emotions; rather, it surrounds that part of us that's struggling with kindness and care and gives us a real sense of being heard so we can feel safe and not alone with our uncomfortable emotions.

Self-empathy works best if you slow down and don't use it as a "spot treatment," as many beginners do. In our busy lives, we used to see self-empathy as something to do quickly when we were feeling upset. Thinking we needed some self-empathy, we would identify how we were feeling and what we were needing, hoping we would feel better right away. After thirty seconds of what was mistaken for empathic presence, we were left feeling dissatisfied. Ironically, we would never give empathy to other people in this way but for some reason we treated self-empathy differently. At some point, it dawned on us that what we needed to do was empathize with ourselves the same way we would empathize with others. We began this practice by talking to ourselves. At first, it felt strange and uncomfortable. We were embarrassed to share this practice until we realized that everyone talks to themselves, but those voices are usually just critical voices. *"I am so stupid." "What was I thinking?" "Why did I do that?"* Sound familiar?

Instead of beating ourselves up that way, why not talk to ourselves with kindness and empathy? Ultimately, the most common reason for self-empathy not "working" is that people don't spend time just being with themselves in the moment connecting with their unmet needs. Instead, they move too fast towards resolution in an effort to try to feel better. Empathizing with other people means letting go of any desired outcome, and with self-empathy we want to show up in that same way. Making time and space to be with yourself without an agenda allows for Life Is Wonderful!

Matt's story

Once I normalized talking to myself, I began to look forward to it. I would savor the time in the car with myself, slowing down and making space for what my body was feeling, what emotions were coming up, and what I was needing. I would breathe and pause and listen. I would even imagine I was talking to "Matt" in front of me, empathizing with him, as that helped me (at first, I found it easier to empathize with other people than with myself). Eventually this became more natural and I found it helped with my mindfulness practice. I could just fall back into talking to myself.

I further noticed that talking to myself out loud when I felt triggered or angry with the kids was comforting to them as it gave them an idea of what was going on inside of me.

I had no idea I had such a wonderful empathy buddy right inside of me.

We know our self-empathy guesses are in alignment with our emotional experience when our bodies start to relax in response to those guesses. Just as the eyes are thought of as the window into a person's soul, bodies are the window into a person's inner experience. Feelings, emotions, and moods are typically linked to distinct bodily sensations, even if on a subtle level. By slowing down and becoming more attuned to our bodies, we move toward a better understanding of what's happening in our inner world. It starts by placing our attention on the feelings and sensations in our bodies, locating areas of tension, constriction or contraction, and then listening from the heart. When we listen to ourselves in this way, we open ourselves to the possibility of discovering what need or value lies beneath. Our bodies have an intelligence of their own, and the primary way they communicate with us is through feelings, sensations, and emotions. Even when the message is not apparent to us, our body talk is intelligent and makes sense, providing us the opportunity to realign body and mind through an understanding of what need or value is at the source.

Our bodies, thus, are our ultimate guide in terms of how to best connect. There are certain ways of relating to ourselves that may increase our likelihood of gaining this connection. For example, it's helpful to state our self-empathy ponderings as questions. The intention is to ask ourselves about our current experience, not tell ourselves what it is. There are times when we don't know what we're feeling and needing until our bodies relax around a particular guess. This is the power of guessing, as it provides a process of truly wandering into our experience so that we feel heard, understood, and accompanied.

Another way we connect to our experiences is by focusing our self-empathy ponderings on what our experience is like. We can guess about certain bodily sensations we notice (tension in the traps or shoulders, constriction in the throat, heaviness in the chest, or tightness in the stomach) and ask ourselves whether that sensation has any connection to a specific need that isn't being met. Or we can inquire more deeply into our emotions or moods of the experience. We can ask ourselves whether we'd like some acknowledgement or understanding for what we're going through emotionally—especially around the difficulty of our experience.

We can also notice and name the story we're telling ourselves about our situation and wonder how it is contributing to our emotional experience. Sometimes it can be connecting to give ourselves the opportunity to dream about what outcome we'd love to see regardless of how crazy or unrealistic they may be. Dreaming about the best-case scenario and how our needs could be met is another way to empathize with ourselves. In the above example of father and son, a possible dream scenario might be something like this:

(Dad's inner voice)

Would you love to spend quality time with your boy in a carefree way? Laughing with him over the smallest things? Or, maybe have a meaningful conversation about what he's currently going through? And wouldn't it be a dream come true if you could effortlessly see his beauty and innocence in every interaction that you have together? Wouldn't it be sweet if you would have such a reservoir of warmth, love, compassion, and care in your heart that regardless of how he showed up, you could respond in a way that feels good?

The more we can connect with ourselves in this tender, honest, and creative way, the more warmth, accompaniment, and stability we'll have regardless of our emotional experience. Remember that even though this doesn't necessarily change the outcome of a situation, it can greatly impact how we experience it and how we show up as a result of that perception (which, ironically, might then change the outcome of the situation).

There are times, however, when a part of us might not want to listen to what our bodies are trying to communicate. We might be genuinely uncomfortable about having, or even ashamed to have, certain feelings or emotions. For example, we may be fundamentally uncomfortable with feeling resentful or bitter. We may have a belief that it's petty and thus suppress or distract ourselves from the felt bodily experience we might associate with bitterness or resentment. Or we might have an unwillingness to acknowledge how tight and constricted we get around this person or that situation. Maybe we don't want to admit that we're afraid or we don't want to appear timid. In short, we don't want to think of ourselves or appear to others as weak, petty, selfish, scared, immature, lazy, or incompetent. Further, we may not feel confident enough to handle certain feelings, dreading that opening the door to those feelings might let loose a floodgate that would completely overtake us.

Alona's Story—Part 1

After my dad died, I committed to numbness. No longer did I want to feel loss, pain, sadness, grief, anger, and devastation. On the surface was rage that my father was prematurely taken from us, yet underneath was anguish and fear. These emotions were overpowering. The world became a dangerous place. To love and care meant to be vulnerable to loss. In this state of threat or high alert, my body responded with fight, flight, and freeze. I was fighting to remain numb, worried that if I opened my own Pandora's box, I would never be able to close it. My pain was so deep that I was convinced that if I let myself cry, I would never stop. So, I found myself fleeing from anything that might stimulate emotions and therefore frozen (stuck) in my state. As it happened, I was finishing up medical school at the time and the environment did not allow for weakness of any kind. As a result, I "soldiered up" even more, completely suppressing my authentic self, afraid of being perceived as incompetent, inferior, or frail.

In this state, whether consciously or not, I was unable to recognize signals from my body. But the messages were there loud and clear. My chest regularly felt constricted and tight. I was having chronic gastrointestinal issues including bloating, distention, pain, diarrhea, and eventually bleeding. My sleep was erratic, not providing rest and rejuvenation. I felt regularly tired. In an effort to "wake me up," my body was not just talking to me, it was screaming at me.

There are many reasons why we might disregard the messages of our body. Most however, stem from our need to protect ourselves and/or our loved ones. But what are we truly protecting ourselves from? Sometimes it seems like we're trying to protect ourselves from certain people, circumstances, places, or memories. On a more fundamental level, what we're trying to avoid, sometimes at all costs, is how we might feel or what emotions we might have in their presence. We are afraid of our feelings. This aversion is understandable, and to varying degrees, we have all wanted to avoid certain feelings at various times. So how do we honor that part of us which deeply longs for self-connection, self-acceptance, and growth when another part wants to run for the hills?

It comes down to this question: Are we tired of running? Maybe we're not. And that's okay because that's where we are at the moment. But if we are tired of running, then we can stop, turn around, and simply dip our toes in the emotional water we've been trying to avoid. Learning to swim begins by getting our feet wet. Similarly, transformation begins as we slowly face what we feel. We can be motivated by the dream of becoming more comfortable in our own skin, listening to the subtle messages of our body when we feel safe enough and brave enough. If we practice listening to our bodies when they whisper, then, at some point, we may be strong enough to hear them when they scream.

Alona's Story—Part 2

For two years I soldiered on, suppressing and repressing. At this point, I had become completely disconnected from my body and any sensations or feelings it might be having. I even went so far as to ignore the symptoms I was having, pretending they weren't there.

Then one day, sitting in the ICU, writing a patient note, I looked up to see someone sitting directly across from me. He must have seen the exhaustion on my face as he asked me how I was feeling. Having no idea how I was feeling, I looked at him with a blank expression. His response was immediate empathy for how late it was and how draining the ICU could be. The look on his face was so compassionate, his eyes so warm and kind, and his words genuinely caring. I was completely caught off guard and, surprisingly, shared that I was indeed tired and the day in the ICU was extremely challenging. This was the first time in two years that I opened up to anyone, and much less a total stranger.

Going home that night, the experience stayed with me—a testament to the power of empathy. Needless to say, the person I had met was Matt, and the impact of his empathic presence seemed to be the jolt I needed to start shifting. What I now realize is that, in that moment in the ICU, Matt provided me with a sense of safety. That message of safety felt so real, so tender, and so wonderful. It was just enough to have me wanting more. I realized I did want to feel, because feeling nothing meant that I protected myself from the bad but could never feel the good. My fear, my anger, my sadness—they were all still there. What shifted was realizing that to have joy in my life meant also accepting the sorrow. To feel healthy required me to stop ignoring and start paying attention to my body and the messages it was sharing with me. And to heal necessitated that I learn to run towards rather than away from my feelings. This is not easy, and the learning for me continues, but it is absolutely worth it!

Sometimes there's a fear that if we listen to our feelings, emotions, or bodily sensations, then we'll have to do something about it. We'll have to face something that in reality we don't have the strength or desire to face. Instead, we conclude, why bother listening to a voice that we don't have the strength or desire to heed? What we don't realize is that our bodies don't necessarily need action but rather just need to be heard and understood. We can give our bodies this gift when we connect our felt bodily experience to the need or value we perceived as unmet. In this sense, our body's experience can serve as a warning light—an alarm—letting us know a need was perceived as unmet. When we connect that felt bodily experience to the need, the alarm often stops and, incredibly, our bodies find relaxation and peace. That is true even if the actual situation remains unresolved, because what our bodies need to feel peace is more often simply self-connection, not resolution.

The next time a person or a situation comes to mind with an eerie, icky, uneasy, crampy, or gloomy sensation, rather than disregard it, lean into it. Feel it. Consider what need or value may have gone unmet with the person or situation. For example, if it's with a person, it could be that your need to be understood wasn't met. Maybe when you last expressed yourself to that person, he or she took it the wrong way. That feeling you have might be letting you know how much you wanted to be understood and how that didn't happen. Or maybe what comes to mind is a recent situation that left you feeling uneasy. Perhaps your felt bodily experience is letting you know that your needs for power and competence in that moment weren't met in a way that you would have liked.

The practice here is to feel the feelings and make guesses toward ourselves as to what the unmet needs or values might be. We know our guesses are correct when we feel our body relax around the guess. Suppose you notice a tight sensation in the back of your throat and heat in your face as you collect dirty dishes scattered around the house. Your guess might look like, "Are you feeling a little bitter right now because you want more cooperation and support in taking care of the house?" If that guess resonates, your body will soften into it and relax. If the guess missed the mark, keep trying.

It can also be the case that after successfully connecting the felt bodily sensation to a need, we may begin to feel sadness or mourning over the unmet need. This is common and natural. Holding space for that sadness by naming it and allowing it to be there continues to support a path of self-connection and a way to be truly comfortable in our own skin. For example, in the situation above, it may look like connecting to the sadness of not having the support and cooperation you so desire. What's helpful to note is that even if there's mourning to be had, it's a sadness accompanied by a quality of peace that's grounding. It's from that place of peace and self-connection where we can choose whether or not we want to resolve or change anything. Often, we will find that by simply connecting what we're feeling to our perceived unmet need, we can achieve peace of mind.

Understanding and connecting to our needs and values moment-by-moment is a powerful, spiritual practice. It not only allows us to see ourselves more compassionately, it strengthens a deeper degree of self-connection and can help us to better meet our needs. For example, let's say we are walking toward a person whom we admire, intending to make conversation, and we realize that what we want at that moment is acceptance. We may still feel overly excited, nervous, or worried, but there would be more purpose behind our approach. Alternatively, upon realizing that our need for acceptance is driving us toward conversation with this person, we may abort the mission! Trying to meet a need for acceptance with someone we don't know very well may no longer seem worth it.

Or let's say we find ourselves wanting warmth and closeness. In this case, we might turn to someone with whom spending time meets those needs. Whatever the case may be, we can be very intentional with our strategies and actions when we're clear on what we want, need, or value. That brings a level of clarity and purpose that is satisfying and self-connecting, regardless of whether our strategies work out. In fact, when our strategies don't succeed, at least in the way we intended them to, we can use that information to help us understand whether the failure was due to a faulty strategy or to misidentification of the nature of our underlying need.

All human beings, to varying degrees, long for their needs to be met—including needs around understanding, growth, inspiration, self-connection, transcendence, meaning, purpose, beauty, compassion, interconnection, presence, warmth, and love. Some choose to meet these needs through their religion or through faith-based communities. Studies show that *"... religious involvement and spirituality are associated with better health outcomes, including greater longevity, coping skills, and health-related quality of life (even during terminal illness) and less anxiety, depression, and suicide."*[2] This makes sense, given that religious communities offer material and emotional support, focus on health-promoting states of mind like gratitude and compassion, and promote moderation or abstinence with respect to substances that could compromise health and well-being.

On the other hand, the aforementioned needs can be met just as well outside of a religious context. For example, many find connecting to nature deeply fulfilling. Others enjoy the creation and appreciation of art, music, food, or literature. Connecting deeply with friends and family is another way. And then for some, exercise, hiking, playing sports, or watching sports with others are sublime outlets for the energy of life. Meaning, purpose, and compassion can be met through caring for others or through humanitarian efforts and environmental stewardship. And needs for presence, awareness, growth, equanimity, peace of mind, and self-transcendence are touched for many through practices such as mindfulness and meditation, without any affiliation to their religious roots. Regardless of how we meet these universally shared needs, whether it's within a religious context or not, knowing that we have them and intentionally finding a way to meet them on a regular basis allows the energy of life to flow through us in satisfying ways.

The spiritual practice as presented in this chapter is about consciously flowing with the energy of needs. This includes connecting to them and meeting them in ways that are not at the expense of other needs we have, the needs of others, or the health of our planet. As just discussed, we can meet these universal needs in radically different contexts. But there's a deeper lesson to be had here: an individual can meet one particular need in many different ways. In other words, we can have different strategies to meet the same need. The freedom and power that can come from this realization shouldn't be understated.

Let's use a need for stimulation as an example. There are many different ways we satisfy our need for stimulation throughout our day. Some of us find it in our work. Others, in hobbies and recreation. And still others, with family and friends. We can find it through music, literature, sports, and exercise.

Do these strategies always meet the need for stimulation? No. When we are distracted or preoccupied, our connection with family and friends can be superficial and over-stimulating. Or when we work out while feeling sluggish, maybe the only needs met are health and consistency. Sometimes the strategies we have to meet certain needs fit the bill, but sometimes they don't. For this reason, keeping ourselves open to the many different ways we can meet the same need is important. The point is that nothing stays the same. And while strategies come and go, the universal needs will always be there. Learning to hold a loose grip on our strategies helps us continue to evolve and grow.

When we become attached to certain strategies for meeting our needs, we run the risk of deep disappointment, anger, conflict, and frustration. To think that only this person, that place, or this thing can meet our needs is not just inaccurate; more tragically, it's a recipe for suffering. This is not to diminish the significance that certain people, places, or things can have for us. But it is important to make the distinction that, while we may have preferred strategies (people, places, things we particularly enjoy), they are not our only strategies. Albert Einstein said, "If you always do what you always did, you will always get what you always got." The spiritual principle here is to not lose sight of the reality that our needs can often be met in more than one way. Learning to separate our need from the strategy we use is part of our spiritual path. The more deeply we realize that, the more free, powerful, and creative we become.

CHAPTER 16

Natural World

Pillar 9

"In every walk with nature one receives
far more than he seeks."

—JOHN MUIR

WHAT DO WE MEAN by natural?
Innate or natural behavior is behavior that is hardwired within us. Natural instincts and reflexes include our survival instinct, reproductive instinct, and social instinct. Our survival instinct incorporates behaviors such as eating, drinking, seeking shelter, and avoidance of danger (jerking our hands back from a hot surface or running from a bear). These are all intended to help preserve our life and health. Similarly, we have an innate instinct to preserve and propagate our species. This is our reproductive instinct that drives us to find mates, have children, and prioritize protecting those offspring for the future survival of the species. Less well known might be our natural social instinct: a desire to belong and be accepted, connected, and empowered. This instinct facilitates achievement of the needs associated with the other two, as it helps with self-preservation and survival (there's safety in numbers) and increases our chances of finding a mate and reproducing.

Atop our natural instincts are reactions that, through repetition, can become habitual—conditioned responses. Whether thoughts or behaviors, they are developed over time and can occur automatically or subconsciously. Often, they involve a cue or context, the actual behavior, and a reward to reinforce the behavior. The cure or context may be a time of day (first thing in the morning: brushing teeth, coffee, breakfast), location (work: hop on email; gym: begin regular exercise routine), person (slow down if in front of police car, wave to a neighbor), or prior stimulus/activity (pull to the side when hearing a siren, check your phone when hearing a ping). Habits are reinforced by a reward, usually resulting in a sensation of pleasure, accomplishment, ease, or relief. They occur automatically and thereby free up the thinking part of our brain to allow more room and space to be involved in other things.

Habits do not always promote health, however. And when we get into a "bad" habit such as eating ice cream late at night (an action that meets some needs at the expense of others), it can be challenging to break. This is primarily so because they occur automatically and hence require conscious efforts to interrupt and stop. Ending an old habit and forming a new one requires mindfulness.

To break a habit, you first need to have awareness of the behavior. If you don't know you are doing it, you won't know you want to make a change. This is not just about cognitive knowledge; it is also about sensations. Often, we feel something isn't quite right before we know why. The same goes for our habits. We may notice feeling tired, sluggish, and uncomfortably full when heading to bed before we connect that sensation to the "ice cream at night" habit.

Next, you need to identify any triggers that might set off the behavior. Maybe you feel hungry at night because you haven't eaten enough during the day? Or could it be that you feel bored, stressed, anxious, depressed, or angry? Every problem is really a solution; in other words, there is always a "good reason" or need you are trying to meet with any action, even those "bad habits," so it is helpful to identify the underlying need. Whatever the reason, knowing what triggers you will help you address your need in other ways. If you are needing sustenance because you didn't have enough food during the day, consider adding more to your meals or having a healthy late-night snack like some fruit. If you are needing regulation, try a meditation session or body scan with breathing. If you are feeling lonely, try connecting to a friend or family member. If you are depressed about going to a job you don't like in the morning, maybe some self-connection around needs for more meaning and purpose would be satisfying. The takeaway is that once you notice what triggers you, you can work on expanding the strategies you use to meet your needs. Over time, and with reinforcement, the new behaviors will become habitual.

Another way to break a habit is to create a competing one. A competing habit brings consciousness to the decision process and ideally makes the old habit more difficult or less desirable. For example, if you are a snoozer and love hitting that snooze button in the mornings, move your alarm to the other side of the room. Now you actively have to get up and out of bed to press snooze. Or if you are the night-eating ice cream lover, don't have ice cream readily available in your freezer. Instead, have a healthy and delicious dessert such as frozen fruit or a nut and date truffle. When faced with going out to buy ice cream or conveniently having the healthy dessert in your freezer, most likely you will pick the latter.

Our natural and habitual behaviors are how we relate to ourselves, each other, and the world around us. Habits are essentially the neural pathways our brain creates to allow us to perform activities of daily living with as little mental bandwidth or attention as possible. For example, the first time you learned to ride a bike, you had to really concentrate, but eventually you created a set of neural pathways or habitual behaviors that allowed you to ride a bike and balance without any thought or attention. Understanding this helps us see that much of what we do is habit arising from our responses to our surroundings. As such, we have agency in what those habits look like, whether they are best serving us in the present moment, and what type of greater impact they may have.

Sadly, although it is a natural desire and instinct, we have strayed from caring about each other and our planet. Still, caring for the world around us and the people in it is part of our basic instinct for self-preservation and survival. It enhances our social connection and preserves our resources, directly increasing our chances for procreation and survival of the species.

In this case, what is natural may not be comfortable because of what has become habitual. Some of the habits we have developed may feel comfortable despite their not serving us, or, even worse, their resulting in disconnection and harm. The comfort and familiarity we feel gives us an illusion of safety that we want to preserve, primarily by resisting change—even when that change is intended to get us closer to our natural state.

In essence, the balance has been tipped toward destructive behavior and habits over protective ones. For example, our natural instinct is to be social and contribute to each other, enhancing our survival as a species. However, the habits arising out of the daily grind have us living in a scarcity mentality that encourages isolation, competition, and antagonism. Rather than hunting and gathering for the tribe, we amass as much as we can for ourselves. Instead of trusting in friends, family, and work relationships, we relate to them with suspicion, ready to discard those relationships at any time. When it comes to supporting our natural world, we choose driving alone over carpooling, creating waste over reusing and recycling, and our favorite foods over more eco-friendly foods. Overcoming these thoughts and behaviors may initially feel cumbersome and undesirable, which is why we often resist making changes.

The good news is that bad habits can be broken. The more we practice incorporating new thoughts and behaviors, the more these become habitual and feel natural. While such thoughts and behaviors initially involve conscious awareness, planning, and intentional effort, over time, this way of thinking and being becomes more and more automatic and effortless.

It is likely clear why this would be beneficial for our self-care as well as our relationships, but why should we care about the greater impact? Reconnecting to the natural world is fundamental to human health, well-being, spirit, and survival—that's why. In his book *The Nature Principle*, author Richard Louv defined the concept of "Nature Deficit Disorder" or NDD as "an atrophied awareness, a diminished ability to find meaning in the life that surrounds us, whatever form it takes." This disconnection from nature comes at a cost that directly impacts our own health, as well as that of the society and environment around us.[1]

Being in nature, on the other hand—sitting on a beach, hiking a mountain, viewing a beautiful landscape—reduces anger, fear, and stress, while increasing pleasant feelings such as calmness, relaxation, and joy. Research confirms that contact with nature reduces aggression and violence. Areas lacking trees, grass, and buildings with greenery see more aggression, more violence, and higher levels of mental fatigue.[2] Furthermore, being outdoors has been shown to improve mood, increase relaxation, reduce anger and anxiety, relieve depression, and improve sleep. In fact, studies have shown that exercising in nature, even in short amounts, improves self-esteem and mood, with the presence of bodies of water having even greater impact.[3]

Exposure to nature promotes "lower concentrations of cortisol, lower pulse rate, lower blood pressure, greater parasympathetic nerve activity, and lower sympathetic nerve activity" compared to city environments.[4] A study looking at roughly 3800 children aged 3-16 found that more exposure to greenness (grass, trees, plants) was associated with having a lower body mass index (BMI). The study concluded that being in nature is a viable approach to preventing childhood obesity.[5]

The benefits don't end there. Studies show that nature increases the value we place on community and close relationships. When in nature, people seem to care more.[6] Interacting together in the natural world facilitates connection and enhances attachment between parents and children. For one thing, shared natural experiences seem to alleviate the stress that both parents and children experience by allowing them to slow down and step away from the daily grind of living in survival mode.[7] Also, family experiences in the outdoors, especially those that are a bit challenging and may require a little work, encourage cooperation and trust. For example, caring for a garden, setting up a campsite, rowing a kayak across a lake all involve cooperation and responsibility. When children see they have something to contribute, they build a stronger sense of self. And adults foster a greater sense of trust and respect in seeing their children's competence, decision-making, and problem-solving abilities.

What becomes apparent is that connecting to the natural world is not just a "nice to have" but actually a "need to have." And until you experience the power and joy of the natural world in your body, it's nearly impossible to comprehend how isolated and lonely you actually feel. The next time you have an opportunity to take inventory, try comparing how you feel before you go for a hike in the woods or walk along the beach to how you feel immediately afterwards. To do this, notice your senses during your adventure: can you smell the air around you, hear the birds chirping or the leaves blowing in the wind, see the trees or the ocean, touch the sand beneath your feet or the flowers along your path? For many of us, engaging with our senses is something we take for granted and often don't pay attention to. Moreover, living in survival mode, devoid of experiences with nature, has served to dull this very important skill set. This may seem insignificant, but sharpening our senses is actually important for our survival. Not only does it help us maintain awareness of our environment (monitoring for safety or danger), but it focuses our attention, increases our concentration, and improves our ability to self-regulate. It does not have to be all or nothing. We don't need to build a cabin in the woods or discard our devices to gain these benefits; we just need to prioritize a connection to nature.

So how do you experience more of the natural world? Ideally you want to get outdoors and be in nature. But even immersing yourself in the natural world while stuck at home or at your desk can be helpful to your health and well-being. Surround yourself with plants, put up pictures of nature, set your screensaver to a beautiful landscape, meditate to outdoor sounds, raise your blinds and open your windows, take a virtual tour of a butterfly garden or your local zoo. The options are abundant, so don't limit your exploration.

If you can get outdoors, do so. Find fun places to visit. Make them closer to home if you have only limited time. Go for a walk, build a garden, have a picnic at the park, take a beach day, join nature clubs in your area. Again, the options are expansive and limited to your imagination and interests.

In addition to being in nature, we have an opportunity to contribute to the protection and conservation of it. Our current reality has us using resources at a rate and extent that we cannot replace, therefore making it unsustainable. In an effort to preserve our environment, we can take steps to change the way we live and eat. Just like any other change we make, we can dive in 100% or make slower, gradual modifications. Small changes made by many are often as impactful, or even more impactful, than big changes made by few. As such, if sustainability resonates with you, start with the things that are easier for you and move along the continuum as you desire.

Here are a few ideas to consider on your journey:

1) Incorporate more whole plant-based foods. Not only are these healthier for you, but it turns out that they are also healthier for the planet. Plant foods, in general, have a significantly lower carbon footprint than animal products. If making more eco-friendly food choices resonates with you, reconfigure your plate to include more fruits, vegetables, whole grains, legumes, and nuts and seeds. Wanting to contribute to the environment but not ready to give up animal foods? Consider limiting rather than eliminating them from your diet. Choosing to eat animal products less often and in smaller quantities moves you along the continuum towards greater sustainability and support of the planet. When possible, try meat alternatives; the varieties available are numerous, so find the ones you like best.

2) Reduce food waste. Food waste leaves a large carbon footprint and unnecessarily burdens landfills. One way to reduce waste is to plan your meals, produce a shopping list of items you truly need, and buy accordingly. You can also consider doubling or tripling your recipes to use up any leftover ingredients. Extra food can be divided into meal-sized portions and frozen for a later date. If you are an avid gardener or considering a garden, start a compost which can provide a natural fertilizer while also lessening the burden on landfills.

3) Reuse and recycle. Benefits of reusing and recycling include conservation of energy and natural resources, lessening of waste, and the reduction of air and water pollution. You can reuse water bottles or shopping bags, switch from plastic to glass, use cloth instead of paper napkins, and have a recycling bin at home.

4) Conserve water. Where you can, be mindful of your water use. Consider turning off the water while you soap dishes or brush teeth, take shorter showers, fix leaks, and use the dishwasher or washing machine only when you have a full load.

5) Plant a tree. Make it your favorite fruit tree and you can reap additional benefits while helping to release oxygen and remove carbon dioxide from the air.

CHAPTER 17

Let's Make Life Wonderful

"For each illness that doctors cure with medicine, they
provoke ten in healthy people by inoculating them
with the virus that is a thousand times more powerful
than any microbe: the idea that one is ill."

—MARCEL PROUST, ~1900

T HE CONVENTIONAL MEDICAL system sets a goal to get you "back to your baseline" or to within normal limits ("WNL"). Often, if this can even be achieved, it is done through medical management, meaning you are treated with pills and procedures. This approach may help decrease your blood pressure, lower your cholesterol, or stabilize your diabetes, but there is minimal improvement in your quality of life, or even, surprisingly, in your risk of overall mortality. In other words, even with those improved numbers, you are still sick. For example, studies show that nearly 75% of patients hospitalized for a heart attack had cholesterol levels that were NOT considered to be high risk. What's more, these conventional treatments tend to revolve around bloodwork results or medical diagnoses while ignoring social and family history. Your treatment plan rarely, if ever, takes into account significant developmental trauma, challenges connecting to family or friends, lack of meaning and purpose in your work, alienation from nature, social isolation and loneliness, or living in survival mode and burning the candle at both ends. The bottom line is that aiming for "within normal limits," or your baseline, is not synonymous with being healthy and falls significantly short of thriving.

At WeHeal, we take a different approach. Our goal is to go beyond wellness to Life is Wonderful. Unlike what commonly happens in most medical visits, we don't start by asking *what's wrong with you*, we start by asking *what does right look like?* What would it take for life to be wonderful? Not perfect and not without ups and downs, but joyful, connected, meaningful, and ultimately wonderful. Many of us have not spent time thinking about who we are authentically, what is alive in us, and how we could feel fulfilled. Yet we believe we have a clear vision of where we want to be and what changes will lead us there. It is for this reason that what we amass (money or status) often turns out not to be what we actually wanted. A common example is people trying to accumulate self-worth by accruing net worth.

We do not, however, discount those things we wish to change. Instead, our desire is to shift the focus by:

1) *Connecting to your "why."* The most effective way to make life-long changes is to truly connect to why we are making them. By this we mean, how do these changes contribute to making life wonderful? To answer this question requires a deeper connection to your authentic self and the needs that you wish to meet. Are you wanting to reverse your heart disease because you have a need for security—a desire to know that you are optimizing your chances to live a long healthy life? Do you want to show up differently in your relationships because you have a need for intimacy, love, and companionship? Would you like to be kinder to yourself because you have a need for care and self-acceptance? Without this clarity, you may be confusing forward motion with progress. Yes, you are making changes, but no, they are not the ones you truly desire for fulfillment, meaning, love, joy, and health.

2) *Connecting to your "why not."* The most compassionate way to make life-long changes is to connect to why we haven't yet made them. So many of us know exactly what we need to do. We may even know why. Some of us might even succeed in making them come about. Yet we struggle to make them stick. There is a reason

this happens. Many of the "problems" we have actually served as solutions for many years. All of the things you say, think, and do were chosen by you because, at some point, they helped you. The catch is that we continue to use these same strategies well beyond their expiration date. What served you as a child, as a teenager, or even two years ago, may not be serving you now. We have discussed how our childhood need for parental acceptance could lead to the strategy of relinquishing our authentic self. After so many years of suppressing and repressing, that strategy can become habitual. But it is not natural and it doesn't have to be so. As adults, we have greater autonomy and agency and can make different choices. That we often don't indicates that we have not tapped into the needs underlying those behavior choices. Or more simply, that we have not had an opportunity to heal.

To focus on our unwanted behaviors or "problems" is like putting a band-aid on a deep cut. You may protect the surface, but you are not reaching the real problem. The band-aid will inevitably not be enough.

At WeHeal, we work with you to identify the underlying needs you are wishing to meet, as well as offer new and effective solutions. More importantly, we empower you with the skills to repeat this process on your own.

Some may come to us with a diagnosis, whether it is heart disease, diabetes, auto-immune conditions (lupus, arthritis, multiple sclerosis), chronic pain, gastrointestinal issues (colitis, irritable bowel, reflux), depression, or anxiety. Our answer at WeHeal is to dig deeper. We believe that many medical conditions can be prevented or reversed, and for those that cannot, there is opportunity to at least improve the quality of life. But this does not happen with wishful thinking, pills, or procedures. It happens by putting in the time and getting the right support.

So, let's make your DR.EA.MS come true by taking three steps: 1) **D**esired **R**eality, 2) **E**nvisioned **A**ctualization and 3) **M**otivating **S**trategies.

1) **Desired Reality:** Your first step is to get clear on what you want, what is "the dream?" To do this successfully means focusing on, and connecting with, the needs or values you would like to start meeting and experiencing. Think positive and think big! What satisfies you? What qualities do you value? What do you like and want more of? What habits are you unhappy with and willing to release? How would you like to show up? Can you contribute in ways that inspire you?

   As you answer these questions, think about what you do want, not what you don't want. If you want quiet, ask for that. Otherwise, you may ask to turn off the television and instead get a trumpet serenade.

   Some examples to consider:
   1. I want to wake up feeling energized.
   2. I want to lose weight and play ball with my daughters.
   3. I want to be healthy and heart disease-free.
   4. I want a partner in life who cares about me and wants to grow together.
   5. I want to love myself and have compassion for all I have endured as well as support and love for all that I will endure.
   6. I want to find meaning and purpose in my work and contribute to society in a meaningful way.
   7. I want to experience inner peace and harmony.
   8. I want to live with integrity and interdependence, focused on connection (with myself and others) above all else.

2) **Envisioned Actualization:** The next step involves experiencing your desired reality right now, as clearly as possible, using all five senses. Quiet your mind (take a few slow exhales and, if you are comfortable, close your eyes) and connect to what it feels like to head in the direction of your new reality. Really envision it happening and try to experience what that would feel like in your body. Imagine it as clearly as possible, with as many details as you can include. Use all five senses to FEEL what life could be like

when your dream is your reality. Do you feel a sense of expansion, ease, and joy?

Some tips for your journey:

1. FEEL, don't think, your answer. Often it is helpful to picture it using images instead of words. However, if you prefer, you can journal instead.

2. Give yourself time to just be and allow the images to surface. This portion of the exercise should not be rushed in an effort to get "the answers." We strongly encourage you to resist this temptation. You are in the process of painting your picture of Life is Wonderful. There is no rush! Stopping it prematurely leaves you with an incomplete image of what your wonderful life could look like.

Example of what you may notice if weight loss is a desire:

1. I am so proud and happy that I am meeting my need for health and losing weight. My clothes are beginning to fit more comfortably. (Take a minute to get an image and sense of how the clothes feel on your body.)

2. I have more energy to engage in activities I enjoy. (Get a sense of waking up and feeling more energy flowing through you or seeing yourself playing in the park with friends and family.)

3. When I look in the mirror, I feel satisfied knowing that I am heading in my desired direction. (See yourself looking in your bathroom mirror, feeling so proud of yourself with a big smile on your face.)

4. I notice an increased confidence, comfort, and calm in my body that expands into and enhances my relationship with my partner. (See you and your partner together, feeling love and care for each other as you connect to a beautiful sense of inner peace.)

3) **Motivating Strategies:** The final step is to come up with specific actions you can take to realize what you have envisioned. It is not

enough to just say you want to exercise. Make these actions clear, present, and doable.

a) Clear: Get clear on your intention for the moment, day, week, or whatever time frame you choose. If you are someone who needs help with accountability, build that into your strategy. For example, pick a consistent time every day for physical fitness. Give yourself a menu of activities to choose from that you would actually enjoy. Set an alarm to remind yourself, and when it goes off, get moving (staying connected to your felt sense of heading towards your desired reality).

b) Present: Your strategy must be something you will do in the present, not in the future. What do you want to say, think, or do right now, at this moment? It's not about running the marathon six months from now. It's about what you are going to do to start moving today (connect to how you would feel as you meet those needs right now).

c) Doable: If your strategy is not doable, it won't get done. It is as simple as that. You cannot start by running six miles. Instead, start by combining a run/walk for thirty minutes today. For some of you, even that might not be doable. The first day might simply be visualizing yourself on a walk (the key is to connect joyfully to something doable, which can't be done if you are trying to force yourself to do something that is not doable).

As you begin to make your DR.EA.MS come true, remember that you will fall off the desired path. We all do. "Mistakes" are an indication that we are trying; they will continue to happen along our journey. Otherwise, we would already be at the destination. If you are not making "mistakes," then you are likely not growing. So, when a mishap occurs, begin by showing yourself some compassion. Remember your self-empathy or seek empathy from a friend. Next, if you can, find gratitude. If not, find acceptance. Mistakes are messages. In fact, at WeHeal we celebrate "mistakes" as opportunities to dive deeper, learning what you like and what you don't like, what is working and what doesn't work. They tell us, as physicians, that we either haven't tapped into your underlying needs or we haven't yet identified the strategies that will work best for you. The good news is that we have a ton of tools, tips, and strategies. The one that is right for you is just a connection away.

Our final take-away for you is that LIFE IS WONDERFUL. Not that you are happy all the time, but rather that you have access to a full range of awareness and emotions that steer you towards a compassionate consciousness—one that honors and supports all universal human needs (not some needs at the expense of others). This experience of harmony and resonance with yourself and the world around you demands a higher level of consciousness and intention. Connection (to self and others) is what stimulates that highly sought-after sense of inner peace. And joy happens as a result of *living* your personal growth journey, not *completing* it. In this state, you understand that there is more to life than avoiding pain and harm. You understand that greed and scarcity are the result of wounding as you strive to heal, and you learn to view the world through a lens of abundance and interdependence. Your life energy leaps beyond the pursuit of safety, to a place where lasting joy, satisfaction, and inner peace is the norm. What this looks like for you is waiting for you to discover and experience. Don't rob yourself of another minute; your time for Life is Wonderful is right now!

It Can Be Different!
Let Us Help You

"Although no one can go back and make
a brand new start, anyone can start from
now and make a brand new ending."

— CARL BARD

This book is a helpful start on your path to Life Is Wonderful; however, if you would like more support to encourage, motivate, and enhance your long-term success, then please reach out to us at:

www.WeHeal.health

We offer a variety of options to tailor and best support your journey towards optimum health and living in a state of Life Is Wonderful. There is no better time than now to get started. We look forward to seeing you soon!

APPENDIX A

Activities to Reduce Stress

Key activities that help put the brakes on your sympathetic nervous system:

- Take full deep NOSE breaths (breathe in through the nose for a count of 4, hold for a count of 7, and blow out through the mouth for a count of 8)
- Alternate nose breathing (inhale and exhale through one nostril, full deep breaths, then repeat using the other nostril)
- Put cold water on your face
- Dance in your living room like a child at a birthday party
- Eye gazing (try staring into a friend or family member's eyes for twenty seconds, sending love and care to each other)
- Hug yourself and rub your upper arms up and down (you can include breathing in and out while you do it)
- Place your hand on your heart and take a deep breath
- Name what you are feeling out loud or write it down (you can do this as expressive writing and tear it up after, if desired)
- Hum, sing, gargle (stimulates your safety brake via the throat)
- Smile for twenty seconds (you can even sit with a pencil or sensory stick in your mouth to stimulate the "smile" muscles)
- Side-to-side stimulation (move your eyes from left to right or alternate tapping your left and right thighs)
- Lean into your thoughts with breath awareness:
  - Don't try to make the thoughts or fear go away, rather use those thoughts to identify the need to send a message of safety. Breathe all the air out that you can and then breathe in all the air that you can to full capacity and repeat. You can agree to do this five times in a row and then notice how you feel.

Agree to do this every time you get an image that stimulates stress or fear or threat. This way you are telling yourself that it is okay to have anxious thoughts but that you will do these five breaths every time you notice them, even if you find that you need to take the five breaths many times in a row. These thoughts simply signal fear and nothing more. It is helpful to do this breathing exercise every time you identify a threatening image or thought so that you start to associate safety and calmness with the experience you are fearing (whether a past experience or future experience). Once you have done these five breaths multiple times in response to the fear your body is signaling through the image or thought, eventually your brain gets bored, as it realizes it is safe and would prefer to put its attention elsewhere. By not trying to make the thought and anxiety go away and replacing it with this "message" of safety through the five full breaths exercise, you are going to make the thought and anxiety dissolve (it is counterintuitive).

- Connect with yourself or others by honing in on feelings and needs that are present in the moment (if alone, try talking them out loud)
- Laugh
- Journal—Engage in Expressive Writing
- Regulate your breathing
  - Deep breathing and alternate nostril breathing are quick tools among many to help regulate the nervous system quickly. The key is to practice these tools and prioritize regulation of your body throughout your day as a regular practice, rather than just waiting for your body to perceive a threat. It is like putting coolant in your car for steady regulation of the engine temperature versus waiting for the engine to overheat and then trying to cool it down.
- Mind the gap—take that pause
  - "Between stimulus and response, there is a space. In that space lies our freedom and our power to choose our response. In our response lies our growth and our happiness."—Viktor Frankl.

If we can take a pause to orient and regulate and check in with ourselves, we can come from a place of intentionality rather than reactivity. In this way, we can take back our power and come from choice. We can choose how we respond and how we show up in the moment.

Appendix B

Essence of WeHeal

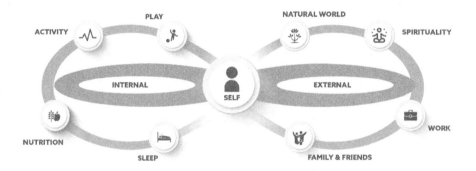

Appendix C

Physiological States and Nine Pillars of the Essence of WeHeal

Physiological State (the basics)

- The physiological state of your body is affected by your perception of threat vs. safety. When your body senses that it is safe, based on its experience of its environment (neuroception) through what it sees, smells, hears, feels, and tastes (rather than you intellectually understanding that you are safe), then it enters an anti-inflammatory state that allows you to rest, digest, and reproduce. However, when the body senses its environment is unsafe or dangerous, then it enters a proinflammatory state to prepare to fight, flee, freeze, and begin damage control.

- The physiological state of threat or high alert is distinctly different and essentially the opposite of the physiological state of safety. Here are just some of the many physiological changes that occur in the different states:

THREAT	SAFETY
PROINFLAMMATORY: cytokines released from cells to address damaged tissues and/or fight invading pathogens.	ANTI-INFLAMMATORY: cytokines released from cells to let the body know it's safe to rest as there's nothing to fight right now.

THREAT	SAFETY
HALT cellular "housekeeping" activities (such as those removing mutated cells that can turn into cancer) to shift resources towards threat neutralization.	CONTINUE cellular "housekeeping" activities (such as those removing mutated cells that can turn into cancer).
Blood shunted AWAY from your viscera and gut to your extremities to support fighting, fleeing, or freezing.	Blood shunted TOWARDS your viscera and gut to your extremities to support rest, digestion, growth, and reproduction.
Blood shunted towards the HINDbrain, INCREASING ability to react quickly, and DECREASING ability to connect or think logically.	Blood shunted towards the FOREbrain, DECREASING reactivity, and INCREASING ability to connect or think logically.
RELEASE of various hormones and neurotransmitters including adrenaline, cortisol, and histamine to support fighting, fleeing, or freezing.	SEQUESTER of hormones and neurotransmitters ordinarily secreted in high amounts during stress (adrenaline, cortisol, and histamine) to support rest, digestion, growth, and reproduction.
Muscles in the face and neck TIGHTEN to portray a DEFENSIVE posture (e.g., anger, fear).	Muscles in the face and neck SOFTEN to portray a CONNECTIVE posture (e.g., happy, peaceful).
Muscle in inner ear and larynx adjust/tune to receive and emit HIGH frequencies of HURT and LOW frequencies of AGGRESSION.	Muscle in inner ear and larynx adjust/tune to preferentially receive and emit NEUTRAL frequencies of CONNECTION.

- Both physiological states are essential for your survival and are extremely helpful when they occur at the appropriate times and with the appropriate duration, magnitude, and frequency. Most chronic disease occurs when we spend too much time in the proinflammatory threat or high alert state and don't balance that with enough quality time in the safety state. We are designed to be in the threat or high alert state for short bursts and then go back into the safety state.
- The state of our environment and how we choose to interact with our environment is what determines if/when we shift from a state of safety to threat and then back to safety. Most chronic disease is the result of, or is affected by, chronically activating the threat or high alert state.
- Anything that affects your perception of safety vs. threat will change your physiological state. This includes affecting the hormones, neurotransmitters, or "biochemical soup" flowing through your body as well as where the blood flows and which muscles and nerves are activated at which times throughout the body.
- Emotional, mental, and spiritual threats trigger the same physiological changes as physical threat, as far as our bodies are concerned.

Life Is Wonderful (the basics)

- Imagine walking through your world experiencing your life as nothing short of wonderful. Not that you are happy all the time, but rather that you have access to a full range of awareness and emotions steering you towards a compassionate consciousness that honors and supports all universal human needs (not some needs at the expense of others).
- This experience of inner peace and resonance with your world demands a higher level of consciousness and intention. In this state, you understand that there is more to life than avoiding pain and harm. You understand that greed and scarcity are the result of

wounding as you strive to heal and view the world through a lens of abundance and interdependence. Your life energy leaps beyond the pursuit of safety, to a place where lasting joy, satisfaction, and inner peace is the norm. We call this state Life Is Wonderful.

- Life Is Wonderful looks different for different people, so you must identify what this state looks like for you, then take action to head in that direction
- It is not about always living in the state of Life Is Wonderful; rather, it is about knowing what the path looks like for you, how to identify when you have fallen off the path, and how to get back on the path as effectively as possible.

Everything we do at WeHeal can be boiled down to helping you optimize the nine pillars of the Essence of WeHeal so that you MAXIMIZE:

- your time in the physiological state of safety (recalibrating your nervous system so that you can respond to the world from a state of safety most effectively), only activating the physiological state of threat or high alert when truly appropriate, supportive, and beneficial to your overall health and well-being.
- your time in the state of Life Is Wonderful, whatever that means to you, so that you can experience a life full of joy, satisfaction, and inner peace.

Nine Pillars of the Essence of WeHeal

- Self
  - When you suppress your feelings and needs to stay attached and in (artificial) harmony with others, you signal to your body that your authentic self is dangerous to share; this triggers the physiological state of threat or high alert. When this happens, we stimulate the proinflammatory responses as described in

the chart above, which in turn supports chronic disease. In addition, you validate the behavior that continues suppressing and repressing, so that you enter an ongoing downward cycle.

- Self-connection to your needs, even if you can't meet them, is the clearest path towards inner peace. Imagine showing up at every moment in your superhero pose as you proudly say to the world, "This is me!" When you can embrace and "expose" all of who you are, Life Is Wonderful.

• Nutrition
  - When your body ingests toxins or poisons, it perceives threat and deploys a host of inflammatory cellular reactions to fight off and eliminate those toxins. If the food we consume is not recognized by the body as our natural fuel, then it will be seen as a toxin or poison, triggering the physiological state of threat or high alert. When this happens, we stimulate the proinflammatory responses as described in the chart above, which in turn supports chronic disease.
  - When we consume food that doesn't weigh us down with salt, fat, sugar, and cholesterol after each meal, our bodies feel nourished, strong, and revitalized, and Life Is Wonderful. When we can eat delicious, natural, health-promoting food until satisfied and feel energized afterwards, Life Is Wonderful.

• Activity
  - When your body doesn't move, it assumes that there must be some threat that is preventing you from being active. Our natural state is to be mobile, so when sedentary, your body will trigger a threat response to try to reverse whatever is preventing our natural level of activity. When this happens, we stimulate the proinflammatory responses as described in the chart above, which in turn supports chronic disease. Once we restore activity in our life, our body will turn off the physiological state of threat or high alert and shift us back to a state of safety.

- Notice how wonderful it feels to stretch and move, compared to how awful it feels to be confined to bed rest. Our natural state is to move and expand with the energy and flow of life, and when we do that, Life Is Wonderful.

- Play
  - Playing, or "being," is about making space to be present without the sense of having to do or accomplish something. When we are in the mindset of having to do something, then we create a sense of pressure and in some cases a sense of danger or anxiety in our bodies around that task not getting accomplished. We can easily identify play, as it entails "being" rather than "doing." What's more, you cannot play and be anxious at the same time. Play can only occur when we are not in a state of threat or high alert. When we play, we are essentially telling our body that all is safe. As far as our body is concerned, the only thing that will limit our natural tendency to play is some sort of "threat," including anything that must be done for fear of consequences. As a result, when we have a "play deficiency" and/or restrict play in our lives (as a result of always "doing"), then we miss out on these opportunities to rest from "doing" and our bodies assume we must accomplish those tasks or something "bad" will happen. This triggers the physiological state of threat or high alert. When this happens, we stimulate the proinflammatory responses as described in the chart above, which in turn supports chronic disease.
  - Imagine yourself just "being," making space in the present moment to allow life to unfold for a bit without trying to make anything happen. The creation and holding of space "to be" instead of "doing" is the key, along with trusting that what will naturally come out of that space will be more wonderful than something you could "force."

    Or imagine playing all of what you loved to do as a child. Observe children—their natural inclination is to play. In fact, it is so important to them that it is hard for them *not* to play.

Everything we work towards can come back to a desire to play in your world with the people you care about. Play doesn't just feel good; it signals to the body that at least in this moment, Life Is Wonderful.

- Sleep
  - Our bodies must sleep. Humans are the only animal on this planet that deliberately interferes with, and restricts, sleep. As far as your body is concerned, the only reason you wouldn't sleep is if it isn't safe to do so. Otherwise, you would always sleep sufficient hours because it is essential to your survival. In other words, if we don't optimize our sleep, our bodies will assume there is some threat preventing us from doing so, triggering the physiological state of threat or high alert as a result. When this happens, we stimulate proinflammatory responses.
  - When you protect your sleep, you tell your body that it matters more than anything else. You also relay to it that it is safe. When you get a full night of restful sleep, notice how wonderful you feel, as if you can accomplish anything. Sleep is the single most effective way to wipe your health slate clean each day. When you rest and restore your body, you set your day in motion to ensure Life Is Wonderful.

- Family/Friends
  - When we are disconnected from our friends and family, we feel a sense of isolation. This experience can be stimulated by: what we Say (how we communicate), how we Think (our beliefs), and/or what we Do (our behavior). Humans are a social species designed to be connected, and when that is lacking, the body perceives that disconnected state as dangerous. As a result, anything that disconnects us from the people we care about will trigger a state of threat or high alert in our bodies. When this happens, we stimulate the proinflammatory responses.
  - When we are connected to our friends and family, we feel a sense of comfort and safety. Beyond that, when our relation-

ships are thriving, we are inspired and feel a sense of hope. It is easy to see how, when our relationships with our family and friends are thriving, Life Is Wonderful.

- Work
  - Some people work at their current job only to make money to survive. When we work in that survival state, we are not doing it for the joy of contributing to society; rather, we are doing it out of fear for our own survival. That fear stimulates a state of threat or high alert in the body. In addition, if our team runs on artificial harmony, it signals to every team member's body that interacting authentically is dangerous. What's more, when we lack meaning and purpose in our lives, we feel further disconnected from those core universal human needs. When our needs go chronically unmet, as can happen in our work life, we can not only experience isolation and despair, but further trigger the threat response in our body. When this happens, we stimulate the proinflammatory responses.
  - Imagine going to a job because it affords you an opportunity to contribute to society in a way that is meaningful to you. Imagine going to a job where your team is authentic and attuned to everyone's needs and is unwilling to sacrifice connection for productivity, and where the new measure of success is effectiveness, not efficiency. When your work is an avenue for you to fulfill your higher purpose, whatever that means to you, Life Is Wonderful.

- Spirituality
  - Being connected to something bigger than yourself is a way to expand your reasons for being in this world. If all you care about is yourself, then the world becomes a small and lonely place. Without faith in something spiritually greater, we can easily live in a state of scarcity and fear. When we feel isolated, self-centered, and alone, our body will experience that as dan-

gerous and trigger a threat response. When this happens, we stimulate the proinflammatory responses.
- Imagine waking up with a sense of inner peace because you know that everything is going to be okay. Whether it is faith in your god or in the universe or in some other source of spiritual connection, you can experience a beautiful sense of security, trust, and inner peace. No matter what happens to you on any given day, being connected to something greater than yourself will ensure that your Life Is Wonderful.

- Natural World
  - Humans are designed to be connected to the natural world. All life forms on this planet are "intended" to be in balance with each other. When this connection is severed or out of balance, then our body perceives that as being the result of something wrong. In other words, only when there is a "problem" would we sever our ties and regular connections to all other life. There is a coregulation of our nervous system that can happen as well when we are in nature and with other life on this planet. As a result, disconnection to the natural world leads our bodies to believe something is wrong and triggers a threat response. When this happens, we stimulate the proinflammatory responses.
  - Imagine spending time "forest bathing," hiking in the mountains, swimming in the ocean, walking on the beach, rafting down a river, looking out at a beautiful landscape, or simply cuddling with your favorite pet. These additional connections to our natural world not only have an impact on our physical, mental, emotional, and spiritual health, they are essential if you want to ensure that your Life Is Wonderful.

Appendix D

Feelings & Needs List—Abbreviated

(For a comprehensive list of feelings & needs please visit www.WeHeal.health)

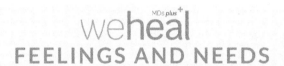

FEELINGS AND NEEDS

PLEASANT FEELINGS	UNPLEASANT FEELINGS
Calm	Angry
Comfortable	Anxious/Nervous
Curious	Confused
Excited	Cranky/Irritable
Grateful	Embarrassed
Happy	Hurt
Hopeful	Impatient
Inspired	Lonely
Proud	Sad
Safe/Secure	Scared
Satisfied	Tired
Warm/Touched	Torn

NEEDS

Acceptance/Belonging	Friendship	Partnership
Appreciation	Health	Reassurance
Care/Consideration	Honesty	Respect
Choice/Autonomy	Hope	Rest
Celebration	Independence	Play
Clarity	Integrity	Peace
Compassion	Joy	Safety/Comfort
Competence	Kindness/Warmth	Security
Connection	Love	Support
Contribution	Mourning	To be Heard/Seen
Ease	Movement	To Matter
Empathy/Presence	Nurturing	Trust
Fairness	Order	Understanding

APPENDIX E

Feelings & Needs List—Kids

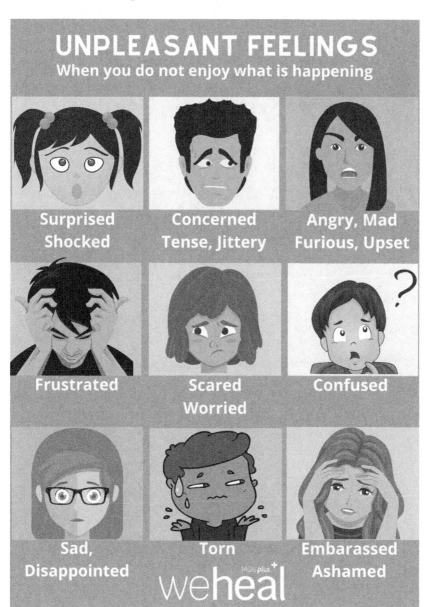

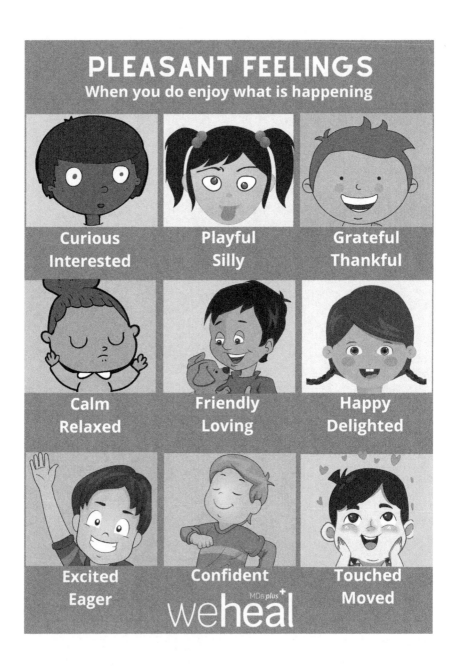

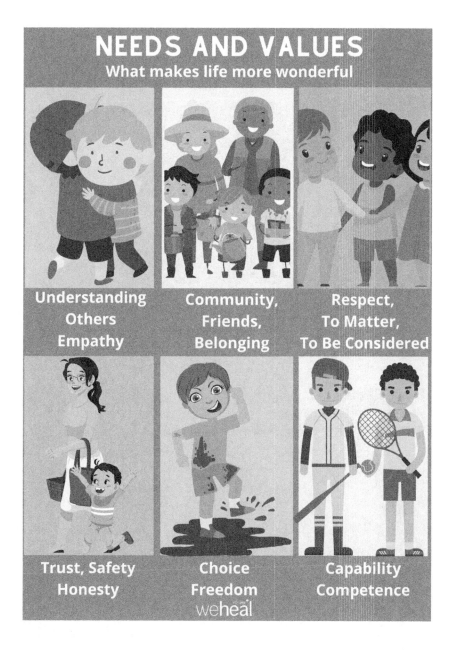

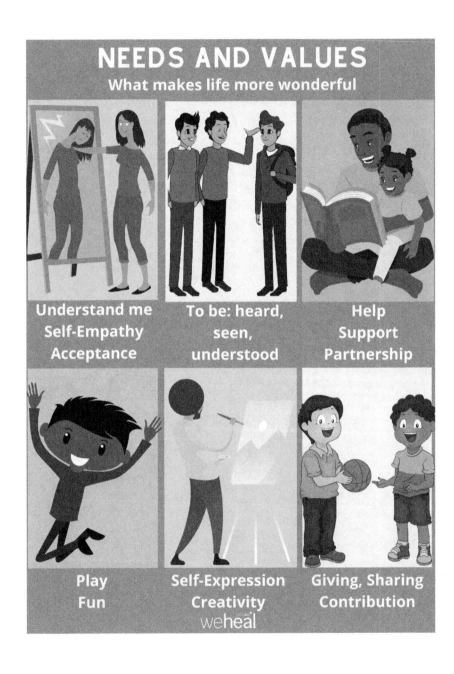

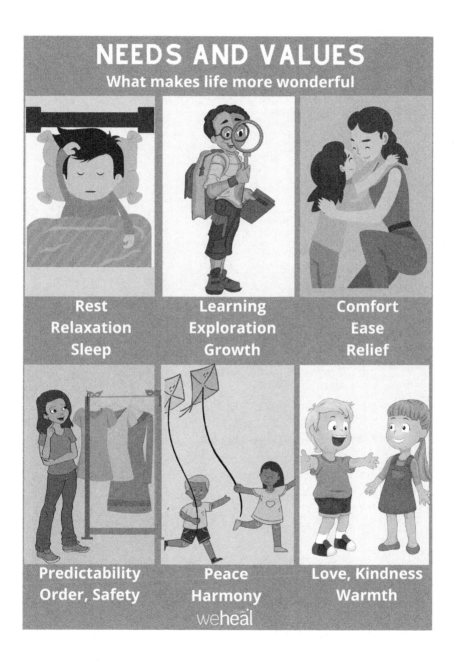

Sensory Experiences List

Sensory Experiences

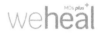

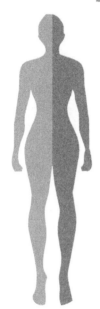

Temperature

Frozen	Burning
Cold	Hot
Cool	Sweaty
Chills	Clammy
Tepid	
Warm	

Motion

Radiating	Twitching
Pulsating	Shaky
Trembling	Pounding
Jumpy	Shivering
Spinning	Fluttering
Aching	Spasming
Vibrating	Throbbing
Paralyzed	Fluid
	Frantic

Spatiality

Tight	Sufoccating
Contracted	Stretching
Tense	Widening
Pressure	Relaxed
Paralyzed	Opening
Closed	Expansive

Weight & Mass

Heavy	Puffy
Full	Thinning
Weighty	Airy
Congested	Light
Dense	Foggy
Bloating	

Substance

Wood	Mud
Metal	Cotton candy
Electricity	Bubbles
Light	Rubber
Air	Water
Iron	Sand
Fire	Fog

Miscellaneous

Numb	Hard
Stinging	Glowing
Prickly	Strong
Damp	Smooth
Neutral	Energized
Sharp	Blocked

Check-In Meter

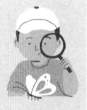

Check-in Meter

10 — My mind and body are jumping all around.

9

8 — My mind is busy and my body is tense.

7

6 — My mind is moving and my body is uncomfortable.

5

4 — My mind is cloudy and my body is softening.

3 — My mind is clearing and my body is calming.

2

1 — My mind and body are calm, peaceful, and open.

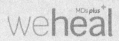

Endnotes

Introduction

1. https://www.cdc.gov/mentalhealth/learn/index.htm
2. https://www.cdc.gov/suicide/facts/disparities-in-suicide.html
3. https://www.cdc.gov/ncbddd/adhd/data.html
4. Ibid.
5. Hojat M, Louis DZ, Markham FW, Wender R, Rabinowitz C, Gonnella JS. Physicians' empathy and clinical outcomes for diabetic patients. *Acad Med.* 2011 Mar; 86(3): 359-64. Doi: 10.1097/ACM.0b013e3182086fe1. PMID: 21248604.
6. Del Canale S, Louis DZ, Maio V, Wang X, Rossi G, Hojat M, Gonnella JS. The relationship between physician empathy and disease complications: an empirical study of primary care physicians and their diabetic patients in Parma, Italy. *Acad Med.* 2012 Sep; 87(9): 1243-9. doi: 10.1097/ ACM.0b013e3182628fbf. PMID: 22836852.
7. Rakel DP, Hoeft TJ, Barrett BP, Chewning BA, Craig BM, Niu M. Practitioner empathy and the duration of the common cold. *Fam Med.* 2009 Jul-Aug; 41(7): 494-501. PMID: 19582635; PMCID: PMC2720820.

Chapter 1

1. Dyer, Wayne W., MD, *The Shift: Taking Your Life from Ambition to Meaning*, Hay House, 2019.

Chapter 2

1. Srivastava S, Tamir M, McGonigal KM, John OP, Gross JJ. The social costs of emotional suppression: a prospective study of the transition to college. *J Pers Soc Psychol.* 2009 Apr; 96(4): 883-97. doi: 10.1037/a0014755. PMID: 19309209; PMCID: PMC4141473; Symonides B, Holas P, Schram M, Śleszycka J, Bogaczewicz A, Gaciong Z. Does the control of negative emotions influence blood pressure control and its variability? *Blood Press.* 2014 Dec; 23(6): 323-9. doi: 10.3109/08037051.2014.901006. Epub 2014 May 1. PMID: 24786662; Lisko, I, Hall, A, Håkansson, K, Neuvonen, E, Kulmala, J, Ngandu, T, Solomon, A and Kivipelto, M. (2020), Does suppressing one's emotions increase the risk of all-cause dementia among older adults? *Alzheimer's Dement.*, 16: e043899. https://doi.org/10.1002/alz.043899.

2. Kraft TL, Pressman SD. Grin and bear it: the influence of manipulated facial expression on the stress response. *Psychol Sci.* 2012; 23(11): 1372-8. doi: 10.1177/0956797612445312. Epub 2012 Sep 24. PMID: 23012270.

3. Zaccaro A, Piarulli A, Laurino M, Garbella E, Menicucci D, Neri B, Gemignani A. How Breath-Control Can Change Your Life: A Systematic Review on Psycho-Physiological Correlates of Slow Breathing. *Front Hum Neurosci.* 2018 Sep 7; 12: 353. doi: 10.3389/fnhum.2018.00353. PMID: 30245619; PMCID: PMC6137615.

Chapter 3

1. "People spend daily average of seven hours online worldwide," TRT WORLD, 15 Feb, 2022, https://www.trtworld.com/life/people-spend-daily-average-of-seven-hours-online-worldwide-54765.

2. Loneliness And The Workplace, 2020 U.S. Report, Cigna, https://www.cigna.com/static/www-cigna-com/docs/about-us/newsroom/studies-and-reports/combatting-loneliness/cigna-2020-loneliness-report.pdf.

3. Holt-Lunstad J, Smith TB, Baker M, Harris T, Stephenson D. Loneliness and social isolation as risk factors for mortality: a meta-analytic review. *Perspect Psychol Sci.* 2015 Mar; 10(2):227-37. doi: 10.1177/1745691614568352. PMID: 25910392.

4. https://www.cdc.gov/aging/publications/features/lonely-older-adults.html.

5. Eisenberger NI, Jarcho JM, Lieberman MD, Naliboff BD. An experimental study of shared sensitivity to physical pain and social rejection. *Pain.* 2006 Dec 15; 126(1-3): 132-8. doi: 10.1016/j.pain.2006.06.024. Epub 2006 Aug 4. PMID: 16890354.

6. Kross, Ethan et al. Social rejection shares somatosensory representations with physical pain. *Proc Natl Acad Sci USA* 2011 March 28, 108 (15) 6270-6275 https://doi.org/10.1073/pnas.1102693108.

Chapter 4

1. Cole SW, Capitanio JP, Chun K, Arevalo JM, Ma J, Cacioppo JT. Myeloid differentiation architecture of leukocyte transcriptome dynamics in perceived social isolation. *Proc Natl Acad Sci USA.* 2015 Dec 8; 112(49): 15142-7. doi: 10.1073/pnas.1514249112. Epub 2015 Nov 23. PMID: 26598672; PMCID: PMC4679065.

2. Pennebaker JW, Beall SK. Confronting a traumatic event: toward an understanding of inhibition and disease. *J Abnorm Psychol.* 1986 Aug; 95(3): 274-81. doi: 10.1037/0021-843x.95.3.274. PMID: 3745650.

3. Pitkala KH, Routasalo P, Kautiainen H, Tilvis RS. Effects of psychosocial group rehabilitation on health, use of health care services, and mortality of older persons suffering from loneliness: a randomized, controlled trial. *J Gerontol A Biol Sci Med Sci.* 2009 Jul; 64(7): 792-800. doi: 10.1093/gerona/glp011. Epub 2009 Feb 17. PMID: 19223606.

4. Del Canale S, Louis DZ, Maio V, Wang X, Rossi G, Hojat M, Gonnella JS. The relationship between physician empathy and disease complications: an empirical study of primary care physicians and their diabetic patients in Parma, Italy. *Acad Med.* 2012 Sep; 87(9): 1243-9. doi: 10.1097/ACM.0b013e3182628fbf. PMID: 22836852.

5. Hojat M, Louis DZ, Markham FW, Wender R, Rabinowitz C, Gonnella JS. Physicians' empathy and clinical outcomes for diabetic patients. *Acad Med.* 2011 Mar; 86(3): 359-64. doi: 10.1097/ACM.0b013e3182086fe1. PMID: 21248604.

6. Steven R Anderson, Morgan Gianola, Natalia A Medina, Jenna M Perry, Tor D Wager, Elizabeth A Reynolds Losin. Doctor trustworthiness influences pain and its neural correlates in virtual medical interactions, *Cerebral Cortex*, 2022; bhac281, https://doi.org/10.1093/cercor/bhac281.

Chapter 5

1. https://www.cdc.gov/media/releases/2016/p0215-enough-sleep.html.

2. McCarthy, Niall, Americans Are Tired Most Of The Week, Statista, June 8, 2015, https://www.statista.com/chart/3534/americans-are-tired-most-of-the-week.

3. Trampe D, Quoidbach J, Taquet M (2015) Emotions in Everyday Life. *PLoS ONE* 10(12): e0145450. https://doi.org/10.1371/journal.pone.0145450.

4. U.S. Department of Health and Human Services and U.S. Department of Agriculture. 2015-2020 Dietary Guidelines for Americans. 8th Edition. December 2015. Available at: http://health.gov/dietaryguidelines/2015/guidelines/.

5. https://health.gov/our-work/nutrition-physical-activity/presidents-council.

6. Renner, Ben. Survey: Quarter of Americans feel they have no one to confide in. StudyFinds, May 27, 2019, https://studyfinds.org/survey-quarter-americans-have-no-one-confide/.

7. Achor S, Reece A, Kellerman GR, and Robichaux A, 9 Out of 10 People Are Willing to Earn Less Money to Do More-Meaningful Work, *Harvard Business Review*, Nov 6, 2018; Stieg, Cory, You're spending your free time wrong—here's what to do to be happier and more successful, *Make It*, Nov 6, 2019.

Chapter 6

1. https://www.cdc.gov/vitalsigns/aces/index.html.

2. Zelaya CE, Dahlhamer JM, Lucas JW, Connor EM. Chronic pain and high-impact chronic pain among U.S. adults, 2019. *NCHS Data Brief*, no 390. Hyattsville, MD: National Center for Health Statistics. 2020.

3. Daneshjou K, Jafarieh H, Raaeskarami SR. Congenital Insensitivity to Pain and Anhydrosis (CIPA) Syndrome; A Report of 4 Cases. *Iran J Pediatr.* 2012 Sep; 22(3): 412-6. PMID: 23400697; PMCID: PMC3564101.

4. Ashar YK, Gordon A, Schubiner H, Uipi C, Knight K, Anderson Z, Carlisle J, Polisky L, Geuter S, Flood TF, Kragel PA, Dimidjian S, Lumley MA, Wager TD. Effect of Pain Reprocessing Therapy vs. Placebo and Usual Care for Patients With Chronic Back Pain: A Randomized Clinical Trial. *JAMA*

Psychiatry. 2022 Jan 1; 79(1): 13-23. doi: 10.1001/jamapsychiatry.2021.2669. PMID: 34586357; PMCID: PMC8482298.

Chapter 7

1. https://health.clevelandclinic.org/what-happens-to-your-body-during-the-fight-or-flight-response/; Kozlowska K, Walker P, McLean L, Carrive P. Fear and the Defense Cascade: Clinical Implications and Management. *Harv Rev Psychiatry.* 2015 Jul-Aug; 23(4): 263-87. doi: 10.1097/HRP.0000000000000065. PMID: 26062169; PMCID: PMC4495877.

2. Aljoscha Dreisoerner, Nina M. Junker, Wolff Schlotz, Julia Heimrich, Svenja Bloemeke, Beate Ditzen, Rolf van Dick. Self-soothing touch and being hugged reduce cortisol responses to stress: A randomized controlled trial on stress, physical touch, and social identity. *Comprehensive Psychoneuroendocrinology,* Volume 8, 2021, 100091, ISSN 2666-4976, https://doi.org/10.1016/j.cpnec.2021.100091.

Chapter 8

1. Schecter A, Cramer P, Boggess K, Stanley J, Päpke O, Olson J, Silver A, Schmitz M. Intake of dioxins and related compounds from food in the U.S. population. *J Toxicol Environ Health A.* 2001 May 11; 63(1): 1-18. doi: 10.1080/152873901750128326. PMID: 11346131.

2. Baden MY, Liu G, Satija A, Li Y, Sun Q, Fung TT, Rimm EB, Willett WC, Hu FB, Bhupathiraju SN. Changes in Plant-Based Diet Quality and Total and Cause-Specific Mortality. *Circulation.* 2019 Sep 17; 140(12): 979-991. Doi: 10.1161/CIRCULATIONAHA.119.041014. Epub 2019 Aug 12. PMID: 31401846; PMCID: PMC6746589.

3. Mazidi M, Katsiki N, Mikhailidis DP, Sattar N, Banach M. Lower carbohydrate diets and all-cause and cause-specific mortality: a population-based cohort study and pooling of prospective studies. Eur Heart J. 2019 Sep 7; 40(34): 2870-2879. doi: 10.1093/eurheartj/ehz174. PMID: 31004146.

4. https://health.gov/our-work/nutrition-physical-activity/dietary-guidelines/previous-dietary-guidelines/2015.

5. https://www.cdc.gov/heartdisease/facts.htm.

6. https://www.worldhealth.net/news/one_in_three_us_children_born_in_2000_wi/, referencing: JAMA 2003; 290: 1884-1890.

7. Ning H, Labarthe DR, Shay CM, Daniels SR, Hou L, Van Horn L, Lloyd-Jones DM. Status of cardiovascular health in US children up to 11 years of age: the National Health and Nutrition Examination Surveys 2003-2010. *Circ Cardiovasc Qual Outcomes.* 2015 Mar; 8(2): 164-71. doi: 10.1161/CIRCOUTCOMES.114.001274. PMID: 25782775.

8. https://www.cdc.gov/nchs/fastats/obesity-overweight.htm.

9. Key TJ. Diet, insulin-like growth factor-1 and cancer risk. *Proc Nutr Soc.* 2011 May 3: 1-4. doi: 10.1017/S0029665111000127. Epub ahead of print. PMID: 21557887.

10. Larsson SC, Michaëlsson K, Burgess S. IGF-1 and cardiometabolic diseases: a Mendelian randomisation study. *Diabetologia.* 2020 Sep; 63(9): 1775-1782. doi: 10.1007/s00125-020-05190-9. Epub 2020 Jun 16. PMID: 32548700; PMCID: PMC7406523; Berkey CS, Rockett HR, Willett WC, Colditz GA. Milk, dairy fat, dietary calcium, and weight gain: a longitudinal study of adolescents. *Arch Pediatr Adolesc Med.* 2005 Jun; 159(6): 543-50. doi: 10.1001/archpedi.159.6.543. PMID: 15939853.

11. National Institutes of Health Office of Dietary Supplements. (2022). Iron Fact Sheet for Consumers [Fact sheet]. https://ods.od.nih.gov/pdf/factsheets/Iron-Consumer.pdf; Niederau C, Strohmeyer G, Stremmel W. Epidemiology, clinical spectrum and prognosis of hemochromatosis. Adv Exp Med Biol. 1994; 356: 293-302. doi: 10.1007/978-1-4615-2554-7_31. PMID: 7887234.

12. Bolland MJ, Barber PA, Doughty RN, Mason B, Horne A, Ames R, Gamble GD, Grey A, Reid IR. Vascular events in healthy older women receiving calcium supplementation: randomised controlled trial. BMJ. 2008 Feb 2; 336(7638): 262-6. doi: 10.1136/bmj.39440.525752.BE. Epub 2008 Jan 15. PMID: 18198394; PMCID: PMC2222999; National Institutes of Health Office of Dietary Supplements. (2022). Calcium Fact Sheet for Consumers [Fact sheet]. https://ods.od.nih.gov/pdf/factsheets/Calcium-Consumer.pdf.

13. National Institutes of Health Office of Dietary Supplements. (2020). Magnesium Fact Sheet for Consumers [Fact sheet]. https://ods.od.nih.gov/pdf/factsheets/Magnesium-Consumer.pdf.

Chapter 9

1. Robwera, Nicole F. "Americans Sit More Than Anytime In History And It's Literally Killing Us," *Forbes*, March 6, 2019, https://www.forbes.com/sites/nicolefisher/2019/03/06/americans-sit-more-than-anytime-in-history-and-its-literally-killing-us/.

2. Gibala MJ, Little JP, Macdonald MJ, Hawley JA. Physiological adaptations to low-volume, high-intensity interval training in health and disease. *J Physiol.* 2012 Mar 1; 590(5): 1077-84. doi: 10.1113/jphysiol.2011.224725. Epub 2012 Jan 30. PMID: 22289907; PMCID: PMC3381816.

3. Choi KW, Chen CY, Stein MB, Klimentidis YC, Wang MJ, Koenen KC, Smoller JW. Major Depressive Disorder Working Group of the Psychiatric Genomics Consortium. Assessment of Bidirectional Relationships Between Physical Activity and Depression Among Adults: A 2-Sample Mendelian Randomization Study. *JAMA Psychiatry.* 2019 Apr 1; 76(4): 399-408. doi: 10.1001/jamapsychiatry.2018.4175. PMID: 30673066; PMCID: PMC6450288.

4. https://www.apa.org/topics/exercise-fitness/stress.

5. Caplin A, Chen FS, Beauchamp MR, Puterman E. The effects of exercise intensity on the cortisol response to a subsequent acute psychosocial stressor. *Psychoneuroendocrinology.* 2021 Sep;131:105336. doi: 10.1016/j.psyneuen.2021.105336. Epub 2021 Jun 18. PMID: 34175558.; Hartescu I, Morgan K, Stevinson CD. Increased physical activity improves sleep and mood outcomes in inactive people with insomnia: a randomized controlled trial. *J Sleep Res.* 2015 Oct; 24(5): 526-34. doi: 10.1111/jsr.12297. Epub 2015 Apr 21. PMID: 25903450.; Driver HS, Taylor SR. Exercise and sleep. *Sleep Med Rev.* 2000 Aug; 4(4): 387-402. doi: 10.1053/smrv.2000.0110. PMID: 12531177.; Childs E, de Wit H. Regular exercise is associated with emotional resilience to acute stress in healthy adults. Front Physiol. 2014 May 1; 5: 161. doi: 10.3389/fphys.2014.00161. PMID: 24822048; PMCID: PMC4013452.

6. Dall PM, Ellis SLH, Ellis BM, Grant PM, Colyer A, Gee NR, Granat MH, Mills DS. The influence of dog ownership on objective measures of free-living physical activity and sedentary behaviour in community-dwelling older adults: a longitudinal case-controlled study. *BMC Public Health.* 2017 Jun 9; 17(1): 496. doi: 10.1186/s12889-017-4422-5. PMID: 28595596; PMCID: PMC5465590.

7. https://www.hhs.gov/fitness/resource-center/facts-and-statistics/index.
html; U.S. Department of Health and Human Services. Physical Activity
Guidelines for Americans, 2nd edition. Washington, DC: U.S. Department of
Health and Human Services; 2018.

8. https://www.helpguide.org/harvard/whats-the-best-exercise-plan-
for-me.htm?pdf=14955.

9. https://www.health.harvard.edu/staying-healthy/benefits-of-flexibility-
exercises.

Chapter 10

1. Brown, B. The Gifts of Imperfection, Hazelden Information & Educational
Services (2010).

2. Diamond MC. Response of the brain to enrichment. *An Acad Bras
Cienc.* 2001 Jun; 73(2): 211-20. English, Portuguese. doi: 10.1590/s0001-
37652001000200006. PMID: 11404783.; Kentner AC, Lambert KG, Han-
nan AJ, Donaldson ST. Editorial: Environmental Enrichment: Enhancing Neural Plasticity, Resilience, and Repair. *Front Behav Neurosci.* 2019
Apr 16; 13: 75. doi: 10.3389/fnbeh.2019.00075. PMID: 31057374; PMCID:
PMC6477072.

3. Yenigun, Sami, Play Doesn't End With Childhood: Why Adults Need Recess,
Too, Aug. 6, 2014 https://www.npr.org/sections/ed/2014/08/06/336360521/
play-doesnt-end-with-childhood-why-adults-need-recess-too
(accessed 2/7/23).

4. Stuart L. Brown (2014) Consequences of Play Deprivation. *Scholarpedia*,
9(5): 30449.

5. Yenigun, S., op cit.

6. Lee, Wendy, People spend more time on mobile devices than TV, firm says,
L.A. Times, June 5, 2019; U.S. Department of Health and Human Services.
Physical Activity Guidelines for Americans, 2nd edition. Washington, DC:
U.S. Department of Health and Human Services; 2018.

7. https://eric.ed.gov/?id=ED524739.

8. https://www.unicef.org/press-releases/more-half-young-children-
deprived-play-and-early-learning-activities-their-fathers.

9. https://www.psychologicalscience.org/news/minds-business/playing-up-the-benefits-of-play-at-work.html.

10. Brown, Stuart (2009). *Play: How it Shapes the Brain, Opens the Imagination, and Invigorates the Soul.* Penguin Group, Kindle edition, p. 40.

11. Gordon NS, Burke S, Akil H, Watson SJ, Panksepp J. Socially-induced brain 'fertilization': play promotes brain derived neurotrophic factor transcription in the amygdala and dorsolateral frontal cortex in juvenile rats. *Neurosci Lett.* 2003 Apr 24; 341(1): 17-20. doi: 10.1016/s0304-3940(03)00158-7. PMID: 12676333.

12. Verghese J. et al, Leisure activities and the risk of dementia in the elderly. N Engl J Med. 2003 Jun 19; 348(25): 2508-16. doi: 10.1056/NEJMoa022252. PMID: 12815136.

13. Stanford School of Medicine, "Building 'Generation Play': Addressing the Crisis of Inactivity Among America's Children," 2007; Hirsh-Pasek et al, A Mandate for Playful Learning in Preschool: Presenting the Evidence, (2008), Oxford University Press; Wang S, Aamodt S. Play, stress, and the learning brain. Cerebrum. 2012 Sep; 2012: 12. Epub 2012 Sep 24. PMID: 23447798; PMCID: PMC3574776.

14. Strauss RS, Rodzilsky D, Burack G, Colin M. Psychosocial correlates of physical activity in healthy children. *Arch Pediatr Adolesc Med.* 2001 Aug; 155(8): 897-902. doi: 10.1001/archpedi.155.8.897. PMID: 11483116.

15. Yenigun, S., op cit.

Chapter 11

1. Fulgoni VL 3rd, Keast DR, Lieberman HR. Trends in intake and sources of caffeine in the diets of US adults: 2001-2010. *Am J Clin Nutr.* 2015 May;101(5):1081-7. doi: 10.3945/ajcn.113.080077. Epub 2015 Apr 1. PMID: 25832334.

2. WHO technical meeting on sleep and health, 22-24 Jan., 2004, Bonn, Germany, https://www.ilo.org/wcmsp5/groups/public/---ed_protect/---protrav/---safework/documents/publication/wcms_118388.pdf.

3. Chattu VK, Manzar MD, Kumary S, Burman D, Spence DW, Pandi-Perumal SR. The Global Problem of Insufficient Sleep and Its Serious Public

Health Implications. Healthcare (Basel). 2018 Dec 20; 7(1): 1. doi: 10.3390/healthcare7010001. PMID: 30577441; PMCID: PMC6473877.

4. Smith, Dana G., Lack of sleep looks the same as severe anxiety in the brain. *Popular Science*, Nov. 26, 2018, https://www.popsci.com/sleep-deprivation-brain-activity/.

5. Kracht CL, Chaput JP, Martin CK, Champagne CM, Katzmarzyk PT, Staiano AE. Associations of Sleep with Food Cravings, Diet, and Obesity in Adolescence. *Nutrients*. 2019 Nov 30; 11(12): 2899. doi: 10.3390/nu11122899. PMID: 31801259; PMCID: PMC6950738.; Greer SM, Goldstein AN, Walker MP. The impact of sleep deprivation on food desire in the human brain. *Nat Commun*. 2013; 4: 2259. doi: 10.1038/ncomms3259. PMID: 23922121; PMCID: PMC3763921.

6. https://one.nhtsa.gov/people/injury/drowsy_driving1/survey-distractive03/drowsy.htm.

7. https://www.cdc.gov/media/releases/2016/p0215-enough-sleep.html.

8. Kripke DF. Mortality Risk of Hypnotics: Strengths and Limits of Evidence. *Drug Saf*. 2016 Feb; 39(2): 93-107. doi: 10.1007/s40264-015-0362-0. PMID: 26563222.

Chapter 12

1. House JS, Landis KR, Umberson D. Social relationships and health. *Science*. 1988 Jul 29; 241(4865): 540-5. doi: 10.1126/science.3399889. PMID: 3399889. https://pubmed.ncbi.nlm.nih.gov/3399889/.

2. Rosenberg, M. B., *Nonviolent communication: a language of life*. (2015) 3rd edition, PuddleDancer Press.

3. https://www.nytimes.com/1930/11/09/archives/religion-and-science.html.

4. https://www.nonviolentcommunication.com/learn-nonviolent-communication/nvc-sex/ (accessed 2/7/23).

Chapter 14

1. Lieberman MD, Eisenberger NI, Crockett MJ, Tom SM, Pfeifer JH, Way BM. Putting feelings into words: affect labeling disrupts amygdala activity

in response to affective stimuli. *Psychol Sci.* 2007 May; 18(5): 421-8. doi: 10.1111/j.1467-9280.2007.01916.x. PMID: 17576282.

Chapter 15

1. Peyton, Sarah, *Your Resonant Self* (2017), W. W. Norton & Company, p. XXV.

2. Mueller PS, Plevak DJ, Rummans TA. Religious involvement, spirituality, and medicine: implications for clinical practice. *Mayo Clin Proc.* 2001 Dec; 76(12): 1225-35. doi: 10.4065/76.12.1225. PMID: 11761504.

Chapter 16

1. Louv, Richard. *The Nature Principle: Reconnecting with Life in a Virtual Age*, Algonquin Books, Kindle Edition, p. 11.

2. Kuo, F. E., & Sullivan, W. C. (2001). Aggression and Violence in the Inner City: Effects of Environment via Mental Fatigue. *Environment and Behavior*, 33(4), 543-571. https://doi.org/10.1177/00139160121973124; Kuo, F. E., & Sullivan, W. C. (2001). Environment and Crime in the Inner City: Does Vegetation Reduce Crime? *Environment and Behavior*, 33(3), 343-367. https://doi.org/10.1177/0013916501333002.

3. Barton, Jo and Pretty, Jules. What is the Best Dose of Nature and Green Exercise for Improving Mental Health? A Multi-Study Analysis, *Environ. Sci. Technol.* 2010, 44, 10, 3947-3955, March 25, 2010.

4. Park BJ, Tsunetsugu Y, Kasetani T, Kagawa T, Miyazaki Y. The physiological effects of Shinrin-yoku (taking in the forest atmosphere or forest bathing): evidence from field experiments in 24 forests across Japan. *Environ Health Prev Med.* 2010 Jan; 15(1): 18-26. doi: 10.1007/s12199-009-0086-9. PMID: 19568835; PMCID: PMC2793346.

5. Bell JF, Wilson JS, Liu GC. Neighborhood greenness and 2-year changes in body mass index of children and youth. *Am J Prev Med.* 2008 Dec; 35(6): 547-53. doi: 10.1016/j.amepre.2008.07.006. PMID: 19000844; PMCID: PMC2649717.

6. Weinstein N, Przybylski AK, Ryan RM. Can nature make us more caring? Effects of immersion in nature on intrinsic aspirations and gener-

osity. *Pers Soc Psychol Bull.* 2009 Oct; 35(10): 1315-29. doi: 10.1177/0146167209341649. Epub 2009 Aug 5. PMID: 19657048.

7. Erickson, Martha Farrell, PH.D., Shared Nature Experience as a Pathway to Strong Family Bonds, Children & Nature Network, Vol. One, No. 1, https://momenough.com/wp-content/uploads/2011/04/Shared-Nature-Experience-Family-Bonds.pdf.

Acknowledgments

We would like to appreciate the following people who have contributed to this book and to enriching our lives. To Glen Merzer, thank you for offering your expertise and keen eye in editing this book and bringing it to fruition. To Jeff Melton for spending time meticulously proofreading and reviewing. Thank you to our WeHeal team for your belief in our vision and your willingness to take this journey with us. It is so gratifying to work with such a remarkable group of people and to be inspired daily by your competence and care. Thank you Sylvia Haskvitz for reading every word of this book and sharing essential feedback as well as for providing invaluable support as Matt's assessor, teaching and role modeling how to truly "live" NVC. Thank you to LaShelle Lowe-Charde and Michael Dillo for sharing your wisdom and helping to infuse the consciousness of NVC into our being. And finally, thank you to our beautiful and spirited daughters Kylee and Jordan for continuing to hold us accountable to living in a state of Life is Wonderful.

About the Authors

Alona Pulde, MD and Matthew Lederman, MD

Touted as doctors of the future by Dean Ornish, MD, and with their work supported by many experts including Sanjay Gupta, MD, Dr. Alona Pulde and Dr. Matthew Lederman combined conventional Western medicine, Chinese medicine, Lifestyle medicine, Nonviolent Communication, Polyvagal Theory, and Trauma-Informed, Somatic Principles & Pain Reprocessing to create their groundbreaking health paradigm. They have been successful corporate leaders, starred in the life-changing documentary Forks Over Knives, lectured for eCornell, served as adjunct medical school professors and corporate medical advisors, and are NY Times best-selling authors.

Together they have co-authored five books, including The New York Times Bestseller Forks Over Knives Plan, Forks Over Knives Family, and Keep It Simple, Keep It Whole. With John Mackey, co-founder and CEO of Whole Foods Market, they co-authored The Whole Foods Diet and The Whole Foods Cookbook. They consult for companies such as Whole Foods Market and serve on advisory boards for various organizations.

Dr. Alona Pulde, a board-certified practitioner of Acupuncture and Oriental Medicine and Family Medicine Physician, is particularly passionate about supporting clients with nutrition and addressing women's health. Dr. Matthew Lederman is a board-certified Internal Medicine physician and CNVC Certified Trainer of Nonviolent Communication. He is particularly passionate about integrating mind-body health treatment and providing second medical opinions for patients with persistent chronic disease.

After ten years of serving Whole Foods Market as corporate Vice Presidents, helping launch the company's national comprehensive medical and wellness centers, coaching and retreat programs, and integrated hospital and insurance networks, Dr. Pulde and Dr. Lederman moved on to co-found their new venture, WeHeal, which is the culmination of decades of learning and practical experience organized into an easily accessible program that does everything just short of guaranteeing lasting health, joy, and satisfaction in your life.

With Contributions from
Lisa Rice and Mark Ideta

Lisa Rice is a Health Coach and Plant-based Educator. She spent six years on the Whole Foods Medical & Wellness Center and Health Immersion teams. She has been teaching plant-based cooking for decades, working with individuals and groups, on local television and at lifestyle conferences. Lisa holds a Masters in Traditional Asian Medicine from Emperor's College, is a graduate of the Rouxbe Plant-Based Professional Course and the Global College of Natural Medicine, and is a Certified Yoga Instructor through Yoga Works. She worked for over a decade as an acupuncturist, herbalist, and yoga instructor in Los Angeles and Austin. Before she switched careers, Lisa was a record company executive in New York and Los Angeles, working in publicity and marketing on national campaigns for major label recording artists. Lisa's passions are cooking for family and friends, writing, reading, gardening, and sharing her life with her husband David, teenage son Judah and their chicken, canine, and feline children.

Mark Ideta graduated from the University of Southern California, Santa Barbara, and completed his graduate studies at Fuller Theological Seminary in Pasadena. He brings elements of Nonviolent Communication (NVC), Internal Family Systems, and Hakomi to his personal and interpersonal mentorship approach. His passion to heal and serve has inspired a commitment to lifelong learning. Among his extensive accomplishments are an intensive Mindful-Somatic trauma therapy course, a year-long course centered around resonance-based healing, and ongoing training and courses through the NVC Academy. Mark lives with his wife, a registered nurse who's pursuing her master's degree in marriage and family therapy, and with their three boys whom they homeschool.

Printed in Great Britain
by Amazon

26773485R00165